A NEW AGENDA FOR MEDICAL MISSIONS

D. Merrill Ewert, Editor

A MAP International Monograph

A NEW AGENDA FOR MEDICAL MISSIONS
D. Merrill Ewert, Editor

A MAP International Monograph

Special thanks to the Christian Medical Commission for granting permission to use the chapter by David Hilton. An earlier draft of this chapter with the same title appeared in International Review of Mission, Vol. LXXVI, No. 301, 1987, pp. 78-81. Used with permission.

Published in conjunction with MAP International's
12th International Conference on Missionary Medicine
June 1990, St. Simons Island, GA.

Layout & Design - Regina Vergara Art
Cover Design - Randy Taylor
Printed in U.S.A.

Additional copies of this monograph, a listing of publications, or more information on MAP International can be requested from:

MAP International
P.O. Box 50
Brunswick, GA 31521-0050
U.S.A.
(912) 265-6010

Table of Contents

Acknowledgements

I acknowledge with thanks the hard work and strong support of several people in the completion of this book. MAP International president Larry Dixon believed in the idea. Meredith Long helped to conceptualize and launch the project. Dotsey Welliver clarified the presentation of ideas and sharpened the prose. Regina Vergara designed the cover and laid out the book. Tito Vergara pulled everything together and made it happen. Finally, my wife Priscilla demonstrated infinite patience and understanding when household chores were left undone while I concentrated on revising and rewriting the manuscript.

1

A New Agenda for Medical Missions: An Introduction

D. Merrill Ewert, Ph.D.

Since the time of Christ, Christians have felt a responsibility to meet human needs. Next to the concern for life itself, probably none is more important to people than health; their health and the health of those whom they love. This, however, raises a basic question. How can we best show the love of Christ and address the health needs of humankind? That concern is the central focus of this book.

This book is different than some. It does not pretend to give definitive answers to all the problems and issues facing Christians involved in delivering health care services. Instead, it represents a small step in the search for better ways to promote health and show the love of Christ in the world. You are invited to join in this quest for better understanding by reflecting on the presentations and case studies in this volume. You may not agree with everything you read but hopefully will be challenged by the perspectives and experiences presented here.

The authors of the different chapters share several things in common. Each holds a deep, personal faith in Jesus Christ and a commitment to address the needs of the poor and oppressed. Each has invested years of effort in trying to improve the health of the world's poor. All have struggled to personally integrate their faith in Christ with their professional skills and responsibilities in treating disease and promoting health. They speak from long and often painful experience in some of the most remote and difficult places on earth. Some have pioneered the development of creative, new programs. Others have tested and helped refine the basic

The author worked in community development in Zaire with the Mennonite Central Committee and later became Africa Regional Director for MAP International. Currently he is Assistant to the Director of the Billy Graham Center and Associate Professor of Educational Ministries at Wheaton College, teaching courses in community development.

principles of community health development as we know them today. All have agonized in prayer over tough decisions, rejoiced in success and learned through their mistakes and failures. All desire to help people experience physical, social, psychological and spiritual wholeness. In the pages ahead, they share what they have learned, trusting that you will be challenged and encouraged by their experience. This is a book for practitioners, written by practitioners.

We are God's agents on earth and want to be responsible stewards of what we know about health and wholeness. Therefore the purpose of this book is to share the lessons learned in health development and to stimulate further reflection in order that we may all more effectively serve the Kingdom of God through health development. With that as the goal, let us map out the journey.

Atkins begins by comparing the contemporary, western view of health with that held by people in other cultures. The latter, he suggests, comes much closer to the biblical view of health than does the former. Wholeness is social and spiritual as well as physical so the goal of health development activity should be shalom— peace or harmony. This means internal peace, peace with God, harmony with the world and with one's fellows. Given the Christian view of persons created in the image of God with personal and spiritual characteristics, bound up in a physical existence, the Church has a unique opportunity to minister to the needs of others. Christian health care can not only deal with all of these dimensions of life, it can mobilize the community to promote healing and health. It also has an answer to the ultimate question of life after death. However, Atkins concludes, we must replace our western view of health with the biblical view.

Against this backdrop, Van Reken reviews the history of medical missions and the development of health. From the early days of the church to the modern missionary movement, Christians have provided health care to the world's poor. Health development has often been viewed as a means to an end. Over the years, Van Reken shows, medical missions has shifted from delivering health care services to enabling people to address their own health concerns. This change has brought a new health care agenda with new roles for nonprofessionals. It has also meant much closer collaboration with local churches, national governments and community institutions. With Atkins, Van Reken sees the emergence of a holistic view of persons that has led to new attempts to integrate health development with evangelism and discipleship. The church and its institutions have and continue to contribute to the promotion of health and wholeness around the world.

A 1978 international conference on health signaled a new and more comprehensive approach to health development. In spite of the efforts of governments and private agencies, the health needs of many of the world's poor were going unmet. The Alma Ata conference, Mosley suggests, represented a shift in priorities from health care institutions to local communities. This commitment to promoting health at the community level, however, conflicted with western values and medical institutions. Part of the answer, Mosley argues, is to support local communities as they address their own physical, social, economic and spiritual needs.

Unfortunately, policy papers and public pronouncements rarely translate into meaningful practice. The introduction of simple, public health measures led to dramatic improvements in health in the West. Despite the Alma Ata conference and its commitment to primary health care, little actually changed. The problem, according to Shaffer, was that the primary health care movement focused on institutions whereas the key to health lies in the community. Shaffer proposes instead, community-based health care (C-BHC) which seeks to mobilize people at the local level to take specific actions that will improve their own lives. Primarily an educational process, this involves transferring relevant knowledge, motivating better attitudes and encouraging the adoption of better habits. This, however, presupposes a belief in people and their capacity to change. Christians who believe in the transforming power of God, Shaffer concludes, should be at the cutting edge of community health development.

As Atkins suggests in the opening chapter, western medicine brought compartmentalization of life and responsibilities to the Two Thirds World. Health was perceived as the responsibility of health professionals, and evangelism as that of pastors and evangelists. In this book's first case study, Fountain shows how a health development program addressed the physical, social, economic and spiritual needs of people in Vanga, Zaire. In the process of providing health care services, the program strengthened the church and mobilized communities to address their own health care needs. This involvement of the church and local people in an integrated health program influenced national policy as Ministry of Health officials saw a new partnership between government and the mission agency. In addition to demonstrating how God's word can address community problems, the Vanga experience shows how the church can help shape a nation's health development agenda.

Poverty and the lack of access to health care also exist in the West today. The gap between the rich and the poor is widening in North America. In the Mississippi Delta in the southern United States, Boelens found many poor suffering from inadequate health care and high infant mortality. The Luke Society initiated a "total person" program that offered curative health care, health education and helped the needy access government services. The program did not meet every human need but worked within the structure of the community as a catalyst for change. As a result, infant mortality fell dramatically. Mothers learned how to better care for their families and the community experienced an injection of hope. The principles of community-based development, Boelens found, work in the West just as they do in the Two-Thirds World.

A case study by Rowland shows how a Campus Crusade program integrated health development and evangelism in Uganda. The strategy was based on community health evangelists (CHEs) whose training combined disease prevention with evangelism and discipleship. Half of the CHEs' training dealt with health issues. The rest addressed spiritual concerns. The program found that motivated volunteers, guided by the Holy Spirit, brought people to Christ and met the health needs of the community.

At one level, holistic development means finding a strategy that integrates the physical and spiritual needs of people. Operationally, it also involves coordinating the activities of different institutions that share a common goal of improved health. Unfortunately, health care professionals providing curative services often feel threatened by programs that focus on the prevention of disease and the promotion of health. At the same time, those working in prevention at the community level do not always appreciate the significant role played by hospitals, clinics and dispensaries. The polarization that often results is divisive and destructive to ministry.

Tshimika's case study shows how a health development program in southern Zaire successfully integrated the delivery of curative services with community-based prevention and training. The Kajiji hospital served as a referral center, provided technical services to the community and played an important training role. The community health program emphasized disease prevention, followed up on patients after their release from the hospital and helped the hospital improve its service delivery. This coordination began with the adoption of a health care policy and the creation of a structure through which those providing curative services met regularly with those involved in training and community work. The result was a more harmonious relationship between institutions, improved health services, better stewardship of resources and a more consistent Christian witness to the community.

Another concern as we look at the future of the church and health development is the role of indigenous health care practitioners. Long examines the issue of control and influence over the adoption of new health behaviors in Bangladesh by focusing on the experience of LAMB hospital. LAMB hospital provided curative services, operated a nutrition program and trained volunteers to do health education in the community. However, what made the program unique was the relationship that emerged between the project and indigenous medical practitioners in the area. The hospital staff provided training, curative services and disease prevention to "village doctors" and traditional birth attendants who play a significant role in community life. With this training came new skills and additional information regarding the prevention of disease and the promotion of health. The result was an unusual partnership by which the mission hospital addressed local health needs through those persons who exercise control and influence in the community.

Although external agents can provide services, ultimately the health of communities will improve when people take responsibility for their own development. Sometimes an organization's development philosophy makes it impossible to achieve the intended development goals. Crespo tells how a Latin American agency set out to promote health development among the Quechua Indians but doing so with a service-delivery orientation. The project developed an infrastructure for delivery health care services, drawing heavily on outside resources. Success was defined in terms of people using the program's services. Although the people enthusiastically welcomed the health education activities in the project, few changed their behavior in response to what was taught.

The development organization then shifted its emphasis from the delivery of services to the facilitation of change. Project leaders began listening more attentively to community concerns. The educational process shifted from transferring information to asking questions that forced people to examine their own problems. The local community took responsibility for the process of change. This shift from delivering services to facilitating change led people to take action on their own that led to improved health.

This concern with local initiative can be clearly seen in Kaseje's case study from Western Kenya. The Anglican Church planned and implemented a program that significantly improved the health of the Saradidi community. People identified their own needs. Volunteers were trained as village health helpers. People changed their behavior in response to new information; they established kitchen gardens, participated in antenatal clinics, immunized their children, began practicing family planning and implementing hygienic measures around their homes. In addition, the program made health services—first aid, antenatal care, nutrition education, family planning—and agricultural information available in the community. The project succeeded because of the mobilization of local people and community resources. Saradidi is a stellar example of integrated, community- based health development.

These case studies show the significant contribution that Christians have made to international health. In a follow-up essay, Hilton examines the future of medical mission. The future, says Hilton, promises to be as exciting as its past though very different. The West must learn from the experience of the Two-Thirds World that pioneered the basic principles of community health development. The church has a unique opportunity to promote holistic health through the local congregation which can function as a healing community. Examples from around the world clearly show how the gospel can transform not only individuals but communities when

Christians are faithful in addressing physical and spiritual needs. This new health care agenda means new roles for the missionary health professional.

As Third World churches mature, the new missionary frontiers to be crossed may be cultural or economic rather than geographic. Christians in the West must not only address needs in their own backyards but also address the underlying political and economic issues. As people are empowered to take responsibility for their own health, health professionals will be freed from routine treatments to deal with the major problems for which they have been trained. Hilton concludes that as the church becomes the healing community, doctors will move away from functioning as body mechanics toward being facilitators of healing, mediating Christ's healing love to the sick and broken.

De Angulo then brings us back to the meaning of salvation and the nature of the Church. In the midst of political, economic and social crises, God has called the Church to be a redemptive community, restoring people to wholeness. De Angulo challenges us to embrace the Kingdom through holistic evangelism that integrates the proclaimed Word with specific actions that address the basic needs of the poor and oppressed.

And how should Christian health workers address these needs? That is the question we will explore in the pages ahead. Think of this as a dialogue with deeply committed friends who are sharing their ideas in the struggle to find better answers. As you read, identify biblical principles of health development. Reflect on the questions at the end of each chapter. Discuss your answers and debate the issues with someone else—a colleague or co-worker. Identify useful suggestions upon which you can build in your own work, discarding what may not apply. Look for lessons that others have learned. Share your reactions and insights with the authors. This book is only the start of a process. To the journey!

2

What is Health?

Tony Atkins, AM, MB, Ph.D.

The ancient Chinese paid their physicians in a rather unusual way. Doctors received a regular fee as long as their patients were healthy. If a patient fell sick, the doctor would not be paid again until the person was restored to health. This system provided incentives for successful treatment. More revealing, however, was the way in which ancient peoples viewed "health." Clearly, they saw health as something worth paying for, something of value in its own right, something worth preserving, something positive.

A Western View

In the West, we generally view health in negative terms. If we are not ill, we are healthy. It is easy to see how this has happened. Science has made enormous advances over the past hundred years, particularly in the area of human physiology and pathology.

These developments have not only been compatible with but also contributed to our view of humans as complicated machines comprising a host of biochemical and physiological systems in delicate balance and susceptible to disruption. When disturbance occurs in one or more systems the person is "ill." Thus, by inexorable application of scientific analysis, the original view of health has been transposed into a negative search for illness. Instead of employing agents to promote health, we have the doctor who is promoted in our minds as a kind of biological engineer trained to detect and then correct faults in the body machine.

Dr. Atkins served in Sudan as Executive Director for ACROSS, an interdenominational relief and development agency before becoming the technical director for World Vision International's famine relief program in East Africa. The Australian government awarded him the "Order of Australia" in 1987 for his service to international relations and leadership in humanitarian aid. Currently, he is a consultant in the design and evaluation of health care programs.

Inadequacy of the Western View of Health

Most practitioners of Western medicine are burdened by a deep sense of dissatisfaction and by an awareness of the inadequacy of our contemporary attitudes towards health and health care. Many of us who are concerned with establishing health care activities in developing countries do so with a sense of foreboding if not despair, an apprehension that we may be inoculating into highly sensitive societies a very virulent pathogen. We may be responsible for an epidemic of misconceptions as to the nature of health, a disorder already endemic in our own society.

There are many reasons why we have come to look upon contemporary Western medicine as being inadequate.

1. **We have lost our Biblical perspective of health.** Our Western concept of medicine is no longer based upon a Biblical view of "health." The medical profession has lost its Christian foundation. Many of us are only now beginning to understand that contemporary Western medicine represents a serious misunderstanding regarding the nature of health. We need to refocus our attention on what God's Word has to say about health.

2. **Medicine has failed us.** The success of medical science in recent years is dramatic and undisputed. Yet, in a very real sense, this success has concealed our failure to achieve a healthy society. In spite of enormous strides in conquering disease and in making medical services widely available, it nevertheless seems likely that people in our developed countries are as unhealthy today as they were a generation ago. Not only have new diseases emerged, but old diseases have reappeared in forms that are new or unresponsive to effective treatment. Patterns of disease have altered. Yet, since the eradication from Western society of major communicable diseases, there has been little objective improvement in the health of our communities. Despite our advances in medicine we still often hear the West characterized as the "sick" society.

3. **Our medicine is unbearably costly.** Political philosophers presiding at the birth of national health services in Western countries predicted that as a result of free health care, or of universal or widespread health insurance, the general health of such Western nations would improve. It was believed that the cost of such national health services would gradually diminish over the years as a result. Today, this view would be considered extremely naive, even laughable. Budgets for health services are spiraling beyond control. The pursuit of health through the practice of medicine has turned out to be an illusive dream.

4. **Medical care is inequitably distributed.** Contemporary Western health care has become vastly more expensive than we could ever have anticipated. The medical priesthood with its myriad of extraordinarily expensive temples is beyond the means of even the wealthiest countries.

Even in the West, we are forced to make decisions based upon the ability of the patient to pay. There is currently much controversy because physicians are obliged to consider cost in selecting treatments for those who are ill. Inequality of distribution of curative medicine in all its complexity and great expense has become inevitable even in the most affluent countries of the world.

In the underdeveloped world, inequitable distribution of curative medicine is far more pronounced. Most of us have seen the multi-storied monuments erected for the treatment of the urban elite. The government of Ghana, according to Morley in a Christian Medical Commission report, estimated that 40 percent of its health budget went to several hospitals that served around 1 percent of the population (1985: 3). The health needs of ninety percent of the population, Morley continues, had to be met with around 15 percent of the health care budget.

Unfortunately, this is a common problem around the world rather than an exceptional case.

5. **Faulty concept of medicine.** The discovery of a pathogenic virus or bacterium may suggest that a particular health problem has a biological cause. It may appear to argue against a psychological or spiritual component in the state of the patient's welfare. This does not, however, stack up to very profound examination. To attribute to this micro-organism the sole, or at least the predominant, causative role in some incident of ill-health is evidence of an absurdly reductionist approach. To do so is to reduce humankind to the purely physical, devaluing the person. A final explanation of health which is purely physical is based upon a materialistic presupposition about the nature of reality. Medical science can demonstrate the presence of the micro-organism. But science has not begun to explain the collapse of the health of the individual coincident with micro-organismal invasion. To say that we can "heal" by modern medicine reveals the level of our arrogance. Clearly, the human body has vast resources upon which it can draw for healing. At best, a physician is merely adjusting the conditions within the body in order to facilitate natural healing. Every surgeon relies upon that or every major operation would end in fatality.

Those of us involved in health development through the church, particularly in the developing world, should analyze both the reason for and the nature of our medical mission programs. Because we have not adequately examined our theology of mission, many of our medical mission programs have become less than distinctively Christian.

An Holistic View of Health

When the World Health Organization (WHO) was founded in 1948, it advanced a definition of health that must have seemed very provocative to the entrenched and institutionalized medical community of that day. The statement said, "Health is a state of complete physical, mental and social well-being and not merely the absence of disease and infirmity." History has proved that definition to have embraced much truth. Yet it is a truth which we in the West contradict in almost every element of our health care service. Health care professionals in the non-Western world have been instrumental in the increasingly widespread acceptance of this definition of health.

An African View

Traditional concepts of health in indigenous societies are in some ways much more appropriate today. At a conference on health and healing, Appiah-Kube, a Ghanaian church leader, shared his society's concept of health:

"Africans make no distinctions between religion and medicine as is the practice in most Western societies. Most Africans think that health is symptomatic of a correct relationship between people and their environment, which includes their fellow beings and the natural as well as the supernatural world. Health is associated with good, with blessing, with beauty; all that is positively valued in life. Illness, on the other hand, shows that one has fallen out of this delicate balance. Concepts of health in the African framework of culture are far more social than biological; there is more unitary psychosomatic relationship; a reciprocity between mind and matter."

In Africa, the very religious attitude towards health is clearly deeply-rooted and widespread. Health is a very spiritual matter. Prior to the Age of Reason, at least, this similarly spiritual view of health was likewise held in the Western world. But as with so many other features of Western   .
society, our concepts and hence our practices have become secularized. The idea of health being a function of "spirit" as well as of "body" has faded into oblivion. The category of "spirit" is no longer taken seriously, and least of all by many physicians. We live in a mechanistic universe and the human being is a mechanism. Our concept of health has become so distorted as to lead us to treat the person with ill-health as we would a machine gone wrong. But Africa preserves the ancient wisdom that saw humankind as much more than a physical object. The person to the African is a spiritual entity and one's wholeness can be invaded therefore from the realm of the physical or from the realm of the spiritual. And those two dimensions are not readily distinguishable nor is a serious attempt made to draw the distinction. The absurdly reductionist, mechanical and negative concepts expressed in some practices of contemporary Western medicine are both contradictory and incomprehensible to tribal society.

Furthermore, African tribal concepts of health incorporate a recognition that health is a function of *community* and not just of individual body chemistry. It is an indigenous concept that acceptance within and harmony with one's family and society are important elements in the healing of a person and in remaining whole. The community itself may be a preventative medicine. We are well aware of the tremendous contribution of community health activities such as immunizations and sanitation in combating communicable disease. They yield a disproportionately high yield of investment. That "community" has more subtle influences than simply participating in such programs is a concept that we acknowledge in our society but ignore in our medical schools. An industrial manager in a factory or an officer in the military appreciates the relationship between the rate of illness in the group and the morale of the community they comprise.

Additional evidence of the veracity of the holistic view of health as held by tribal peoples can be seen in our recent reawakening to the phenomena of *psychosomatic* influences in almost all disease states. We are beginning again to look for *anxiety*, *stress* and even *guilt* to incorporate in our diagnoses. Yet, these are insights which the African has never forgotten. Illness, from that perspective, has always incorporated elements of *disharmony* with the spirit, the family and village society.

Ironically, in many of the countries of traditional mission activity, tribal people (both Christian and non-Christian alike) have an holistic perception of health which we by virtue of our Western sophistication have lost. The people have a more complete, balanced and integrated concept of health that sophisticated practitioners of Western medicines are now struggling to comprehend. Our arrogance in attempting to influence the development of health care services in such countries is amazing. We may have something to offer but it is far more likely that we have much to learn if health care is to be built upon appropriate and indigenous concepts of health rather than upon our own utterly inappropriate, incomplete and distorted pragmatic perceptions. Christians must take seriously this view of total health. It has so much in common with the Bible's own attitude toward health and has so much in common with the ministry of the Master.

A Biblical View

The Bible's attitude toward health can be understood in two words, which for many Christians today are interpreted in purely spiritual terms. In their original context, they clearly make reference to physical health.

Shalom. The first is the Hebrew word, "shalom," usually translated, "peace." Its Arabic equivalent is the common greeting, "sallam alekum," meaning "peace be to you." The Old Testament meaning of *shalom*, however, is much broader than our English word, "peace." In many places, it could be appropriately translated by the word "health." For the Jews of that day as for many in tribal societies today, health was essentially a positive quality that derived from the fact that people existed in total harmony — in total peace — with their world. This harmony includes one's relationship to nature and to one's fellows. It was internal ("peace of mind," as we would say) but most of all, harmony with God.

In Biblical thought it was enmity with God from which all humankind's disturbances — social, psychological and physical — are derived. It must be for this reason that illness is so often related in the Bible to sin. Speaking on the effect of sin in his life, King David said "my bones wasted away....my strength was sapped" (Psalm 32:3-4 NIV). "There is no peace for the wicked, says God" (Isaiah 48:22 NIV). In the face of sin, there is no shalom — no health — says the Lord.

In the prophets the concept of shalom developed as a kind of integrated wholeness of people at harmony with their environment. It becomes a goal which will only be perfectly fulfilled in the Kingdom of God at the end of the age. The prophesied Messiah is called the Prince of Shalom — the Prince of Peace. One of the bones of contention between the true prophets of the Old Testament, such as Jeremiah, and the false prophets was precisely this issue of health in society — of shalom. The false prophets insisted that shalom — health in society — was unconditional. But Jeremiah insisted that it was dependent upon moral righteousness. He complained about the false prophets, "they dress the wound of my people as if it were not serious. 'Peace, peace,' they say, when there is no peace" (Jeremiah 6:14 NIV). These false prophets are saying "shalom, shalom — health, health" — when there is no health. For Jeremiah the absence of health is a mark of judgement against sin in society.

For the true prophets then there could be no state of complete physical, mental and social well-being of the kind defined by the WHO while people are antagonizing God by their moral failure. To be healed must involve forgiveness and reconciliation between people and God, between people and their neighbors. This is exactly what Jesus claimed to bring. The angel announcing his birth said, "Peace on earth among men." This, those Jewish shepherds understood. Jesus had come to bring with him the Kingdom of God and with it the peace that the world cannot give. This only came when accompanied by the forgiveness of sin and by the removal of guilt.

Salvation. The Greek word for peace conveyed mainly the idea of mental tranquility, and so although it is used in the New Testament, another word which the Greeks understood far better in this connection takes over in prominence. That is the word salvation. The angels again anticipated: "Today in the town of David a Savior has been born to you" (Luke 2:11 NIV). To the Greeks, the word *savior* had clear overtones of the medical world. A sotere could very easily be a physician, someone who delivered you from illness. Very often in the New Testament, the word "to save" is used in just this sense. Repeatedly after healing someone, Jesus says "your faith has healed you" (i.e. Mark 5:34 NIV) but the verb he uses is the word "to save." So salvation in the New Testament did not simply mean that a person would be saved. It meant that someone would be made whole; whole in one's relationship to God, whole in one's relationship to others, whole in one's own mind, freed from the conflicts of pride and guilt and often also whole in body. It was significant when Jesus asked the Jews, "Which is easier: to say to the paralytic, 'Your sins are forgiven' or to say, 'Get up, take your mat and walk?'" (Mark 2:9 NIV). The Jews knew that both things are related, harmony with God and harmony within one's own body. Thus heaven in its fullest expression is a place where there will be no pain and no sickness. It would seem that is why Isaiah, when he was speaking of how the Messiah would come to bear the sins of the world, adds "Surely he took up our infirmities and carried our sorrows...But he was pierced for our transgressions, he was crushed for our iniquities; the punishment that brought us peace was upon him and by his wounds we are healed" (Isaiah 53:4- 5 NIV).

The Person. These observations cause us to reflect further upon the Bible's view of the person. We are creatures in which the worlds of matter and of spirit are contingent. Made of dust, yet we are more than dust. We are also made in the image of God. The spirit and the matter are contingent. Unfortunately, very early in the life of the church, its Biblical foundation was undermined by the introduction of Greek philosophical ideas and in particular Platonic thought which says that although two worlds meet in humankind — the world of matter and the world of spirit — these two are nonetheless separate. Within a sector of Christianity, the subtle influence of this philosophy remains today. The body and the soul have been divided and so they suggest that a person is really a kind of physical machine with a spirit living inside. But that is not what the Bible says. Genesis does not say that God gave man a living soul. It says God *breathed* into him, into his physical nature made out of dust, and he *became* a living soul. In other words, man's personal and spiritual characteristics are inextricably bound up with his physical existence.

What then does the Bible's view of health mean to the Christian? What does it mean to reappraise our attitudes to health and society? How can we achieve a more healthy society? It would seem that any perspective of health that views people as mechanisms, as collections of intricately adjusted biochemical organs, is "sub-Christian."

Shalom/salvation involves not just physical wholeness, but also social and spiritual wholeness embracing the totality of human life. And because it has these social and spiritual dimensions, health is conditional on social and moral as well as medical standards. Because we are fallen creatures, there can really be no health in a total sense except God prepare a way for forgiveness and renewal.

Ultimately, our pursuit of health in society without Christ is futile. So it seems that the Bible's attitude toward health in many ways has a lot in common with the traditional African approach. It is much more compatible with traditional indigenous approaches than with the secularized medicine of the contemporary Western world. This means that committed Christians who serve Scripture in formulating a philosophical basis for their health care activities will emerge with a concept that is not only distinctively Christian, but is also more readily comprehended by non-Western peoples.

The Role of the Church

Given the Biblical perspective of the nature of persons and of the factors impinging upon health, what are the practical implications for the Church?

Salt of the earth. It is interesting to see the Church characterized as the "salt of the earth." By that Jesus undoubtedly intended to convey that the church had a preservative, and antiseptic or sterilizing or hygienic role to play in society. An antiseptic force in a sick world?

Transposed into the Western world environment it is difficult to see such concepts influencing existing structures short of revolution. That would make many of us Christians uncomfortable. Our progress in pursuing pragmatic solutions (in contrast to Christian solutions) to social problems has led us far down the path of commitment to unresponsive institutions which may at their best comply with our wishes but are unlikely to meet our needs. The Christian medical worker in the Western world is entitled to share in at least small measure some of the pathological pessimism into which some have fallen.

What does a Christian view of health have to say to Christians in the church in developing countries? What does it have to say to medical missions standing beside the church? For many years, as Van Reken shows in the third chapter of this volume, medical missions have been providing health care alongside an attempt to heal the spiritual infirmity in humankind. In many cases, medical missions may justifiably be accused of falling into that old trap of separating a ministry to the body from a ministry to the soul.

Medical missions has traditionally been oriented toward curative care in a hospital setting. Does this make it Christian medical work? What makes Christian medical work distinctive? Is it simply secular work performed by Christians?

James McGilvray, former Director of the Christian Medical Commission, suggests:

"Whenever the Church has been loyal and true to its Lord, there have been glorious examples of the application of medicine to the neglected and the outcasts of society...and the willingness to serve in isolated areas where the practice of medicine brings no prestige and very little monetary reward" (McGilvray, 1984: 8).

He continues:

"For the future, the Christian contribution to medicine will primarily be at the point where it reflects and embodies Christ's own teaching, example and judgment. It can make a signal contribution to our understanding about health, extricating it from the narrow confines of medicine where it is now trapped...the Church must also continue to sustain and re-invigorate those Christians who are professional medical workers of whatever kind and enable them not simply to use medical practice as Christians but to use judgment and become agents of change with the system of which they are a part" (McGilvray, 1984: 8).

What is *Christian* health care as distinct from the secular variety? Health care that treats the person as a psychosomatic whole is *Christian* health care; a physical being, a psychological being, a social being and a spiritual being.

Community. These facets of human life that have just been mentioned are not separable and treatable by specialists in their narrow fields. On the contrary, they are interrelated in a highly complex fashion to make us either ill or well, to make society sick or healthy.

Christian health care is health care that works on that presupposition. In practice, Christian health care is going to take very seriously the role of *community* in healing and health. Placing someone in a hospital is surely the course of last resort. The decentralization of health care into small health centers at the village level is much more likely to cater to the total needs of people and therefore to their society than is a more centralized (and remote) hospital.

David Werner's classic book, *Where There is no Doctor*, revolutionized the way many people think about health care (1978). He argued that most health problems can and should be treated at home or in the local community by people trained to look after their own health. The 1978 International Conference on Primary Health Care at Alma-Ata in the USSR labeled this process, primary health care which is:

"Universally accessible to individuals and families in the community by means acceptable to them, through their full participation, and at a cost they can afford. It forms an integral part of both the country's health system, of which it is the nucleus, and of the overall social and economic development of the community."

Not only is that a much cheaper and more effective way of increasing the health of a nation, but to a Christian it is important because it minimizes the social and environmental disorientation consequent upon entering into treatment. The love and acceptance of one's family and society are important elements in healing and in persevering in health. *Community*, it would seem, for a Christian with a Biblical perspective, is very important in Christian medical care. Building small communities which are self-reliant in medical care is important too. And this of course has political and social repercussions which few of us have even begun to consider, let alone examine from a Biblical perspective.

Forgiveness. There is another dimension that Christian health care service offers that other approaches cannot match. For all their achievements in the delivery of health care services to the masses, even nations such as China and Cuba cannot provide it. That is this Biblical insight into the *healing power of forgiveness*. Earlier, we noted that when David failed to confess his sin, he suffered physically. Guilt and its concomitant anxiety and stress are clearly emerging as exceedingly serious factors in the development of ill health in society. Our late awakening to the truth may be excusable for the scientist in us who seeks to see and cultivate the causative agent. It is totally inexcusable in a physician claiming a *Christian* insight. It seems clear that for our own as well as for tribal societies, the achievement of true Christian health care places a demand for more personnel professionally trained as adequately in the area of pastoral care and counseling as they are in clinical medicine.

Training needs to cross these specialist barriers which we have erected between the sacred and the secular. Interdisciplinary study of medicine and psychiatry and social psychology and pastoral theology may be what is needed. In developing countries, there is every prospect that such suitable people may emerge at much less cost and with less effort and trauma out of peoples already identifying with a holistic concept of the spiritual and physical person attuned to and at peace with one's environment.

It is significant to note that Mosaic law placed health care in the hands of Levitical priests—the community health workers (CHW) of their day— who were also able to offer sacrifices for the sins of humankind. This was the same CHW active in God's healing of disease in a community. Now especially in non- western society where the prospect in implementation is most promising, we may be in great error if we are not carefully exploring prospects for encouraging the local church to emerge as a health center. We may be neglecting the enormous potential of the church to contribute toward community health in the fullest sense of the word.

Terminal Care. Finally, there is another area where Church-based health care programs have enormous advantages over the secular. This is clearly evident in seeking solutions to the problem of "terminal care." That is one area where pragmatic health care is proving at best impotent and at worst horrifyingly counter-productive. One of the fascinating uses of *shalom* in the Old Testament is in its application to death. When a righteous person dies, the Hebrew says that person departs in *shalom*. The person departs in peace. One dies in good health. Paradoxical to our way of thinking, for to us health is the constant seeking to evade death. Yet in accordance with the Bible's view of health, one of the marks of the truly whole person is that one is able to die in a state of harmony with others and with oneself and with one's God. Can twentieth century medicine give this?

If Jeremiah were here today and casting about for some false prophets talking about "peace, peace — harmony — health" without relating it to the moral condition of people's souls, he might well find those false prophets wearing white coats and stethoscopes; and of course, just like those false prophets of his own day, completely oblivious to the fact that they were proclaiming "health, health" where there was no health.

Conclusion

The time has come to rethink our approach to health development. Those of us concerned with health development have too often brought our Western view of health and with it inappropriate, expensive health delivery systems that fail to meet the needs of the world's poor. The view of health held by our brothers and sisters in the Two-Thirds World comes much closer to the biblical view of health and wholeness that we have discussed here. The rest of this book will examine some principles of health development and provide case studies showing how they have been applied to practice.

References

McGilvray, James. "The Church and Health: Reflections and Possibilities." *Contact*, The Christian Medical Commission, Number 81, pp. 1-11, 1984.

Morley, David. "The Child's Name is Today." *Contact*, The Christian Medical Commission, Number 86, pp. 1-9, 1985.

Werner, David. *Where There is No Doctor*. Palo Alto: The Hesperian Foundation, 1978.

Questions for Reflection

1. How would you describe a Biblical perspective of health? What Scripture would you use to evaluate your viewpoint?

2. Have you or someone you love been the victim of the inequality of distribution of curative medicine? How did you feel? What does this say about the ability of the western health care system to meet the needs of the poor and oppressed?

3. What would you consider the central elements of a "theology of health development?" What would a health care system based on Biblical principles look like?

4. Can you think of an example where the community contributed to healing and wholeness, apart from any specific medical intervention? What happened? What does this suggest regarding the role of the church in health development?

3

Medical Missions and the Development of Health

David E. Van Reken. M.D.

Missions and Professional Health Care Workers

Historical Overview of Medical Missions

"God had one Son and He was a medical missionary!" With these words mission organizations have challenged medical students to consider careers in missionary medicine. Jesus Christ was a healer frequently moved with compassion by the physical suffering of people he met. Being divine, he was able to instantly cure many of their diseases. He commanded his first-century disciples to teach, to preach, and to heal (Matt. 10:8).

While healings by Christian leaders have markedly decreased since the first century, concern of believers for the sick, destitute, poor, orphans and the outcasts of society has not. Despite vigorous and often bloody persecution, the early Christians showed love to the down-and-out, and with evangelistic zeal spread the Gospel to the far edges of the Roman Empire and beyond. By the end of the third century, approximately ten percent of the Empire's fifty million people were believers.

Between A.D. 300 and 1500 the Church became not only popular, but powerful. Evangelistic fervor decreased and the Church turned to warfare as its means of expansion. Yet some bright spots shone through these dark days of Church history. Home-based hospices and monastery-based hospitals developed in the fourth and fifth centuries in many cities. The Romans had built slave and military hospitals for economic and political considerations. The Church, however, introduced the notion of hospitals as clear expressions of Christian charity.

Formerly a missionary physician in Liberia with SIM International, Dr. Van Reken wrote a history of medical missions while serving as the Billy Graham Center Scholar in Residence at Wheaton College. He is currently Clinical Associate Professor of Pediatrics at the Indiana University School of Medicine.

Far more important than the hospitals themselves, however, Christianity brought a new attitude toward the sick. The church genuinely practiced compassion for the sick and suffering, as taught by Jesus in the story of the good Samaritan. "Whereas disease in the entire course of previous historical development had sharply isolated the sufferer, in Christian times he was actually brought closer to his fellowmen by the fact of his illness" (Sigerist, 1960). A natural outflow of this concept would seem to be medical missions.

With few exceptions, however, no missionary doctors or nurses were sent to the mission field before 1800. Dr. John Thomas (1757-1801), a Christian physician who served the East India Company as a ship's doctor, was the main exception. The physical and spiritual needs of the Indian people moved him deeply. In 1787, he decided to remain in Bengal and minister to their needs. During the next five years he lived in a simple bamboo hut and learned enough of the Bengali language to preach in it. He also ministered to the sick, the hungry, and the naked who came for help.

Later, Thomas returned to England in order to recruit assistance. His appeal to the newly formed Baptist Missionary Society on November 13, 1792, for missionary work in India so moved the committee that he was immediately accepted as their first missionary. A young missionary candidate, William Carey, then volunteered to accompany him to India. In this way, God used Dr. Thomas to call Carey to India in 1793. Over the next 40 years, Carey opened up India for the Gospel as no one else has ever done. Carey's book, *An Enquiry into The Obligations of Christians to Use Means for the Conversion of the Heathen*, ignited the tremendous interest in missions in the early nineteenth century.

The first American missionary physician was Dr. John Scudder who went to Ceylon (now Sri Lanka) in 1819, and later India. His enthusiasm for serving God through missionary medicine led six of his children and four grandchildren to follow in his footsteps. One of the grandchildren, Dr. Ida Scudder, founded the Vellore Christian Medical College and Hospital in India in 1900.

Dr. Peter Parker, the first American missionary physician to China, arrived there in 1834. He established a hospital and became the first surgeon to use anesthesia in China. Along with Dr. Colledge, he developed a program for training Chinese medical students in Western medicine, and co-founded the Medical Society of China.

The year 1841 was a banner one for medical missions. Dr. Peter Parker challenged British audiences with a clear call for medical missionaries while on his way home to America for a furlough. Dr. Abercrombie of Edinburgh founded the Christian Medical Society in response to Dr. Parker's messages. By 1915, CMS operated 54 hospitals worldwide with 4,000 beds. At least 86 missionary physicians, 69 missionary nurses, and

230 indigenous doctors and nurses served in these hospitals (Harding, 1915). Also in 1841, David Livingstone sailed for Capetown, South Africa, beginning his career as a missionary physician.

Livingstone's main accomplishments, however, were not in medicine. His vision opened Africa to trade and education and speeded the end of slavery, something he abhorred. His geographical exploits and botanical observations made him world famous by the time of his death in 1873. His life and death motivated hundreds of missionaries to follow him to Africa.

The idea of doctors and nurses serving on the mission field is recent. In 1850, there were only a dozen missionary doctors. By 1900, there were approximately 650 physicians on the field. The political power of colonial governments, the growing awareness of conditions in poor nations and the increased ability of physicians to actually improve the health of patients contributed to this increase. Mission societies utilized medical personnel to expand their work.

In many countries, missionary medical work was the wedge prying open the door for the other mission efforts. Korea was a sterling example. The first missionary arriving on a passenger ship in 1869 was "bludgeoned to death fifteen minutes after stepping on shore" (Scott, 1983: 10). Several years later a Christian physician, Dr. Horace Allen, won the confidence of the ruler of Korea. Dr. Allen stopped the bleeding from a deep wound in the King's nephew after the local treatments failed. The respect for Dr. Allen which followed permitted the first Presbyterian, Horace Underwood, and the first Methodist, Henry Appenzeller, to enter Korea as missionaries in 1884. Subsequently the laws were changed to allow Korean citizens to become Christians. Dr. Allen later became the first American ambassador to Korea (Hefley, 1971). Today the Christian church in South Korea is considered one of the strongest in the world.

The twentieth-century stimulus for medical missions was triggered by the life and work of Dr. Albert Schweitzer. In the early 1900s, he established a hospital at Lambarene in the West African nation of Gabon. A genius with four earned doctorates (music, philosophy, theology and medicine), he captivated the world's attention by dedicating the last 60 years of his life to serving the poor. This earned him the Nobel Peace Prize in 1952.

The twentieth century saw rapid initial growth in the numbers of doctors and nurses on the mission field, but the numbers have leveled off since 1925. In that year, 1,157 missionary medical doctors served in mission hospitals alongside 614 national physicians. Most of those national physicians were trained at one of the 19 Christian medical colleges offering a full medical course. In 1925, 914 students were enrolled in these schools. Also in 1925, 1,932 nursing students were enrolled in the 66 nursing schools run by missions (World Missionary Atlas, 1925). There were 1,307 missionary physicians in 1932, 828 in 1963, and 1,021 in a count of 59 church or para-church bodies in 1979 (Herschberger and Wingerson, 1979).

Professional Health Care Workers in Missions

Doctors and nurses have not always been welcome members of the mission family. Missions emphasized soul-winning and this was considered to be the responsibility of preachers, teachers and evangelists. Early missionaries were encouraged to learn basic first aid in order to handle their own medical problems in the remote places where they would preach or teach.

In the nineteenth century a few missionary candidates began to study medicine before beginning their mission careers in remote areas of the world. David Livingstone, for example, earned his degree in theology and then studied medicine as part of his preparation for missionary work. He had no intention of becoming a "medical missionary." He planned to serve as a minister just like any ordinary missionary (Walls, 1982: 287). "Hudson Taylor, the founder of the China Inland Mission, and himself a doctor, saw medical missions in similarly strategic terms and consequently advised medical training only for candidates who were too young to go abroad" (Williams, 1985: 275).

During the latter half of the nineteenth century, some mission societies employed doctors to provide medical services to their missionaries on the field. The main impetus for this was the enormous mortality rate among missionaries. The average life expectancy of a new missionary in Africa during the nineteenth century was 8 years (Hefley and Hefley, 1979: 339). Dr. Price estimated that 61% of the 596 deaths among British missionaries before 1910 were preventable with the standard of medical care then available in England (Charles, 1910). While 50 of every 1,000 missionary women died during childbirth on the mission field, only one woman out of a thousand died during delivery in Germany (Olpp, 1932: 159).

The doctor often served only as a hired hand of the mission society. The Church Missionary Society Committee's final instruction to Dr. John Ilott, before he sailed for the West Coast of Africa in 1840 was: "You are not, strictly speaking, a missionary. Your proper place is not to preach the Gospel, but to direct all the energies of your mind and bring to bear your medical experience and skill in endeavoring to alleviate or to prevent the ravages of disease" (Garlick, 1943: 131-132).

Slowly the concept of the use of professional health care workers in missions itself began to dawn. In 1844 Rev. George Smith, on a trip to find openings for mission work in China, came away very impressed with the medical work established by Dr. Peter Parker. He advised his British society to include a health ministry at each station. "This should be," he wrote, "of a decided, unequivocal, primary, and essential Christian character" (Garlick, 1943: 133). Missions began to perceive that health work could be a powerful tool of evangelism, especially in those areas where people resisted the simple message of Jesus Christ. A missionary convention in Liverpool passed a resolution to use medicine to this effect in 1860 (Williams, 1982: 275).

Many missions viewed medical work in utilitarian terms. They referred to it as bait, a magnet, a wedge, or as heavy artillery meant to "soften up the enemy." Medical work was not considered work for real missionaries. As recently as 1876, the Wesleyan Methodist Missionary Society instructed Dr. Langely "that his task was to prepare the people by his medical skills for receiving the instruction of Missionaries, and, therefore, he would not be expected to take the duties of any sick Missionary, or take any active public part in the work of direct evangelization...." (Williams, 1982: 280).

The huge success of Christian health work in areas of great need became obvious to all. Health care workers and their clinics and hospitals were usually overwhelmed by the numbers of patients seeking their service. The mission hospital became the most influential evangelistic center on many mission fields as a "perpetual object lesson of Divine philanthropy" (Williams, 1982: 284).

By the twentieth century, the theology and strategy of missions included health care professionals as vital members of the overall ministry of the mission society or church. The care for physical ailments became accepted as living demonstrations of God's love and concern for hurting people. Instead of being valued less than the truly "spiritual" dimension of mission work, health work became recognized as its necessary expression in a needy world.

Emerging Priorities in Medical Missions

Successive Stages in Health Work

A review of history suggests that medical missions has gone through three stages; doing, teaching, and enabling:

1. **Doing.** The first medical missionaries encountered massive human misery. The health needs of the world's poor, they discovered, were going largely unmet. In the best traditions of Western medicine, these pioneers boldly responded by establishing excellent medical services. In many Third World nations, Christian missions provided a significant percentage of the total health care available. For example, in 1968, church-related hospitals and clinics carried out "43% of the medical work in Tanzania, 40% in Malawi, 34% in Ghana, 26% in Taiwan, 13% in Bangladesh, 12% in Indonesia, 9% in Zaire and 15% in India" (Rasmussen et al., 1980).

2. **Teaching**. Medical missions moved into its second phase when missionary health workers began teaching nationals health care skills. A century ago, some missionaries realized that providing medical services reduced the likelihood of finding long-term, indigenous solutions to local health problems. Nationals must be a part of the solution. For this reason, Drs. Parker and Colledge began training five Chinese medical students in 1845. In India, British medical missionary Dr. Edith Brown founded the Ludhiana Christian Medical College while Dr. Ida Scudder, an American, opened Vellore Christian Medical College. By 1971, Protestant churches and missions operated medical programs in 81 nations. Those programs included more than 1,200 hospitals, four medical colleges, nine schools for physician's assistants and 412 professional schools for nurses (Hefley and Hefley, 1979: 339).

3. **Enabling**. The success of missions in providing health care services and training national health workers led to a third phase called enabling. Enabling involves working with people as equals and in the process empowering them to solve their own problems.

In an enabling relationship, missionaries and national colleagues work together with mutual respect and in submission to each other for the benefit of the community. The process of enabling seeks to promote self-reliance and sustainable indigenous growth and development.

Beyond Doing and Teaching

The concept of enabling emerged from a renewed perspective on what it really means to "help" one's neighbor. How would we want to be helped? We need to give more support and less supervision. Enabling believes that the people themselves are worth far more than any specific goals or work accomplished. While external goals can be reached by force, unless the people have learned something of their condition, learned how to identify their own problems, and experienced success by working out solutions in their own way, ultimately they have not been "helped."

Enabling is hardly new. Medical missionaries have always trained and taught. It is also rare to find missionaries who have not been involved in enabling. An example from northeastern Thailand illustrates the concept. Christian and Missionary Alliance missionaries noticed that nearly one percent of the population suffered from leprosy but that no one did much about it. Being burdened for leprosy patients but untrained in health matters, they contacted Dr. Richard S. Buker, a missionary physician in Thailand, for assistance. Experienced in leprosy work in Burma, he agreed to visit Thailand and give interested missionaries an intensive, crash course on leprosy work. He also agreed to provide them with the necessary medications.

In 1951, Dr. Buker's team treated 12 patients with leprosy. Five years later they had registered 15,000 cases. Five thousand of these leprosy patients received monthly treatments at one of 40 different clinics in the area. Following Dr. Buker's principles, the team established several criteria that villages wanting a clinic were required to meet. Communities were required to provide land and build a grass-roofed structure. Within four months after the clinic began operation, the village itself was required to have an established health committee to dispense the medicine for the patients, keep records, and collect fees. Despite the skepticism of many older missionaries, village people were able to successfully implement the program. Over the next few years, only two of 42 clinics were closed down due to non-compliance, corruption, or mismanagement by the village health committees.

Missionaries moved into the community in order to teach the village health team. Usually within six months after the clinic started, many of the leprosy patients became Christians. When these eager, new Christians wanted to learn more about the Bible and Jesus Christ, the need for further Bible training became obvious. As a result, the Maranatha Bible School (MBS) was established in 1953 as the only four-year Bible school in the world whose students all had leprosy! The school staff and the students raised all their own food on 30 acres of land which they irrigated themselves. UNICEF provided a 400-foot deep well and thus a safe, steady water supply.

The Christians in the villages were encouraged to work hard, own land, build a church building and tithe. The community called a graduate of the MBS to serve as pastor. Thirty indigenous, self-supporting churches emerged from these 40 clinics. Interestingly, while nearly all of the first generation Christians had leprosy only a minority of their children were afflicted. By the third generation leprosy had virtually disappeared.

Testimonies at the Sunday evening services at the Bible school frequently began with the words, "I thank God for my leprosy since through it I found Jesus!" (Kerr, 1982).

Implications for the Future

The experience of the past suggests some implications for the future:

1. **The role of nonprofessionals.** One can promote health without formal, medical training. To some degree health care management has been standardized so that highly effective action can be taken against organic disease through simple treatments administered by nonprofessionals. For example, anyone can mix oral rehydration solution (ORS) as a treatment for diarrhea. Mothers can breast-feed their children instead of using bottled formula. Monthly weighing of children can identify infants at risk from malnutrition, and immunization campaigns can dramatically reduce morbid-

ity and mortality in a region. All of these skills are being applied by uneducated village health care workers around the world. As Hilton says, "if present medical knowledge could be made available to all of the world's people, it would be the greatest advance in the history of medicine" (Searle, 1982: 18).

While health professionals such as Dr. Buker can teach people to solve many of their own health problems at home, other skills can also contribute to improved health. Administrators can help health care teams function together smoothly through good personnel and resource management. Educators can teach health concepts and communication skills. Anthropologists can help the team understand other peoples and develop culturally appropriate programs.

2. **Holistic health care**. We do not treat disease. We treat people who may have diseases so we must remember to practice whole-person health care. The sick person must be viewed as a member of a family and a community as Atkins points out in an earlier chapter of this book. The sick are more than patients with diseased organs; e.g., "the appendix in Room 314." Health care personnel need to be concerned with disorders of the mind as well as the body, with the ill person's psychological and social condition as well as the physical. For Christian health care workers, this concern extends to the patient's spiritual well-being. Health is more than a medical matter.

3. **Focus on health**. The third concern for the future follows and complements the second. Today's focus on health instead of disease means an emphasis upon prevention rather than treatment. People interested in promoting health in developing countries should consider training in Public Health. The pioneer missionary physicians were often surgeons. Today, we need people who can teach, encourage, promote and work with others on the health care team.

The husband-wife team of Drs. Warren and Gretchen Berggren illustrates this trend. After working with Dr. Paul Carlson in Zaire (then called Congo), they studied Public Health at Harvard University and then initiated a primary health care program in Haiti. The program at Albert Schweitzer hospital promoted health education at an average cost of $1.60 per person per year in a certain census tract. Over a five-year period, the infant mortality rate in the target area dropped to one-fourth of the estimated national average. The incidence of deaths from malnutrition, diarrhea and tuberculosis was cut in half, and tetanus deaths were completely eliminated (Berggren, Ewbank and Berggren, 1981).

4. **Collaboration with government efforts**. Future medical missionary efforts must coordinate their activities more closely with national government policies and programs. Clearly, medical missionary work is "temp-

orary and should be continued only until such time as government or other agencies are able to supply the health and medical needs of an area" (Cochrane, 1959).

With the increasing sophistication of the health care sector in developing nations, mission medical programs and resources are best used where the people have the greatest need and the fewest opportunities. The programs will necessarily vary greatly from country to country. In 1985, Togo (West Africa) needed a hospital in a certain location so the Association of Baptists for World Evangelization (ABWE) established one. Other nations need health educators in professional schools or project managers for Primary Health Care programs.

The Christian Medical Commission in Geneva is encouraging missions and governments to cooperate more effectively. They are emphasizing:

"economically feasible and culturally acceptable projects that will provide good health care to the maximum number of people, while permitting each community to participate in the planning and decision-making process. An example is The Lardin Gabas project in Northeast State of Nigeria, where the State government, the local university, the churches, and the community all played an effective role in formulating and implementing the program" (Akerele, Tobizzadeh and McGilvray, 1976: 178).

5. **The National Church.** The ministry of healing will tie in more closely with the total ministry of the national church. Non-Western Christians, as Atkins suggests in this book, often have more holistic views of sickness and health than people from the West. Reflecting the needs of the whole person, indigenous churches can effectively use the ministry of healing to reach out to the community at large with the message of Jesus Christ. However, missions must be careful not to saddle financially struggling churches with the obligations and risks of running a major medical institution.

Unique solutions must be creatively sought. For example, rural pastors are often a community's best health promoters. They have the respect of their communities and have a vested interest in promoting health in this area. The holistic approach of indigenous churches is often more effective in changing attitudes and health behavior than "foreign" mission hospitals. The spiritual and cultural orientation of people are critical in terms of their ability to accept health concepts which require behavioral changes.

6. **Primary Health Care.** An emphasis upon Primary Health Care (PHC) is another new and perhaps the most important trend in missionary health ministries today. In essence, PHC encourages local citizens to become interested, knowledgeable and creatively involved in seeking solutions to their own health problems. Health, from this perspective, is

everyone's responsibility. PHC encourages health care that is readily accessible (available near the home of people who need it), at an affordable cost, and extended in an understandable and acceptable manner. PHC programs are open to everyone in the community and are aimed at preventing and treating the most important diseases occurring in the area.

Initially some missionary physicians worried that PHC could only emerge at the expense of hospital-based medical care. Although tensions exist between some hospital-based and PHC-oriented missionaries, this is clearly changing. Today most health care programs are experiencing improved working relationships between staff involved in providing curative and preventive services. Tshimika's case study from Zaire documents this in another chapter of this book.

In these days of skyrocketing health care costs, the trend towards Primary Health Care is a refreshing breeze. PHC tends to be less costly (but not free!) and pays excellent dividends in improved levels of health. However, such care takes more time and effort to establish since it emerges from the grassroots operation rather than being imposed from the top. The cost and efficacy factors are very important, since the PHC model may be the last chance for improved health for many people in the world's poorest countries. The PHC model is promising because "it turns around the definition of health resources from one which requires massive capital to one which sees potential in every human being. It is the rationalized version of the ancient model of the real self-help organization" (Janzen).

7. **Health and Evangelism**. Missionary health work has an important role in evangelism and church planting. The two functions of medical missions are:

- demonstrating God's love to a needy world
- extending the church of Jesus Christ

We are well reminded "not to think of medical technology or techniques more highly than we ought. What is ultimately most important is how well the missionary health care worker reflects Jesus Christ" (Smalley, 1959: 290). We must remember the overall goals of Christian health work. Never have so many of the world's poor so desperately needed compassionate health care. While serving the poor, the personal witness of God's love in this way leads to spiritual renewal. The experience of the Association of Baptists for World Evangelism is an outstanding example. More than a hundred indigenous churches were established in the Philippines as a result of their work in medical evangelism (Kempton, 1985).

8. **Health Professionals as "Tentmakers."** Opportunities are increasing for Christian health care professionals who want to work as "tentmakers." As professionals with marketable skills, they are obtaining jobs in developing nations which allow them to support themselves financially while sharing Christ and contributing to the development of nations.

In 1984, the *Journal of the American Medical Association* devoted 15 pages to list opportunities for American doctors to work overseas with different organizations. Increasingly, evangelical missions are seconding health care professionals to government and secular institutions. In this way, health needs are being met and a Christian witness established. In some nations where missionaries cannot obtain visas, health professionals have become the initial Christian presence.

Conclusion

The fascinating story of medical missions is still being written. The times are changing. So are the characters, the settings, the methods, and the opportunities. Yet the plot remains constant: the church through medical missions can serve the needy while making disciples in every nation.

These are exciting days in missions as our methods are constantly being revised and our world situation continues to change. Missionary health workers have contributed greatly towards our understanding of various diseases, especially tropical diseases. They have developed innovative, new programs such as primary health care. They are tackling new problems such as health development in urban centers.

Looking back, it is clear that Christian missions — including the health care team — have been successful. Today, we find 13 times more Christians in Asia and Africa than there were in 1900. By the year 2000, the figure will be 34 times as large (Swank, 1979: 207).

Looking ahead, the task is far from over. Now is the time to rededicate ourselves to fulfilling the Great Commission. Unless we redouble our efforts by God's Spirit and begin to penetrate into the large blocks of people in urban, Muslim, Hindu, and Chinese areas, it is estimated that 2.4 billion people will not hear the Gospel by the year 2000 (Swank, 1979).

Christians from a wide variety of professions and with many different skills are needed to work together on today's health care team. As this team witnesses of God's love through the national church in each locality, the physical and spiritual needs of men and women can be addressed.

References

Akerele, O., I. Tabibzadeh and J. McGilvray. "A New Role for Medical Missionaries in Africa." *WHO Chronicle*, Vol 30, 1976, pp. 175-180.

Berggren, W. L., D. C. Ewbank and G. G. Berggren. "Reduction of Mortality in Rural Haiti Through a Primary-Health-Care Program." *New England Journal of Medicine*, Vol. 304, 1981, pp. 1324-1330.

Charles, R. H. "Discussion on Special Factors Influencing the Suitability of Europeans for Life in the Tropics." *British Medical Journal*, Vol. 2, 1910, pp. 859-874.

Cochrane, R. G. *"Changing Functions of Medical Missions."* Address given at First International Convention on Missionary Medicine, Wheaton, Illinois, December, 1959.

Garlick, P. L. *The Wholeness of Man: A Study in the History of Healing.* London: The Highway Press, 1943.

Harding, H. G. *The Story of CMS Medical Missions.* London: Church Missionary Society, 1915.

Hefley, J. C. *The Cross and the Scalpel.* Waco: Word Books, 1971.

Hefley, J. and M. Hefley. *By Their Blood: Christian Martyrs of the 20th Century.* Milford: Mott Media, 1979.

Herschberger, R., and L. Wingersons. "Medicine With a Mission." *Medical World News*, Vol. 20, 1979, pp. 29-36.

Janzen, J. M. *The Development of Health.* Development Monograph Series, No. 8, Mennonite Central Committee, (no date). Mennonite Central Committee, 21 S. 12th Street, Akron, PA 17501.

Kempton, W. W. Personal Communication, August, 1985.

Kerr, Bill. Personal Communication, November, 1986.

Olpp, Prof. "Medical Missions and Their International Relations." In *Modern Medical Missions*, K. W. Braun (ed.). Burlington: Lutheran Literary Board, 1932.

Rasmussen, S., V. Williams, H. Searle, P. John, and C. Taylor. *"The Contribution of North American Christian Missions to Health in Developing Countries."* Unpublished paper, Department of International Health, Johns Hopkins University, July 1980.

Scott, K. M. "Christian Medicine Abroad: A Place for You." *Christian Medical Society Journal*, Vol. 14, No. 3, Fall 1983, pp. 10-13.

Searle, H. G. "Medical Missions Reappraised." *Evangelical Missions Quarterly.* Vol 18, No. 4, 1982, pp. 242-253.

Sigerist, H.E. *On the Sociology of Medicine.* New York: MD Publications, 1960.

Smalley, W. A. "Some Questions About Missionary Medicine." *Practical Anthropology*, Vol 6, No. 2, 1959, pp. 90-95.

Swank, G. O. "The Next Great Advance in Missions." *Evangelical Missions Quarterly*, Vol 15, No. 4, 1979, pp. 206-211.

Walls, A. F. "'The Heavy Artillery of the Missionary Army': The Domestic
    Importance of the Nineteenth Century Medical Missionary." In *The
    Church and Healing*, W. J. Sheils (ed.). Oxford: Basil Blackwell,
    1982.

Williams, C. P. "Healing and Evangelism: The Place of Medicine in the
    Later Victorian Protestant Missionary Thinking." In *The Church and
    Healing*, W. J. Sheils (ed.). Oxford: Basil Blackwell, 1982.

World Missionary Atlas. Edinburgh: Conference of Missionary Societies,
    1925.

Questions for Reflection

1. How has the Christian worldview shaped medical missions?
2. What factors contributed to the significant growth of medical missions in the past?
3. What makes Christian medical work distinctive? Is it something more than just secular work performed by Christians?
4. How does the concept of "enabling" fit into the Christian worldview?
5. How do you see medical missions relate to evangelism and church planting?
6. In view of the changing nature of medical missions, what do you see as the role of the professional health care worker in the years ahead?

4

Principles of Community Health

W. Henry Mosley, M.D., M.P.H.

Introduction

In 1978, national governments joined the World Health Organization and UNICEF in a meeting in Alma Ata, U.S.S.R., to formalize an international consensus on the scope and content of primary health care (PHC) services. As defined in the Alma Ata Conference Declaration, primary health care is very broad and comprehensive. It includes:

- health education
- food supply and nutrition
- water and sanitation
- maternal and child health programs
- immunizations
- prevention and control of locally endemic diseases
- treatment of common diseases and injuries
- provision of essential drugs

Community-based primary health care was hardly a novel concept. As far back as 1946 the Bhore Committee in India proposed the integration of vertical health interventions into a core of comprehensive health services, and all of the elements for community-based programs were well articulated by Maurice King in the book *Medical Care in Developing Countries*, reporting on a symposium in Africa in 1966. By adhering to the Alma Ata Conference Declaration, however, national governments for the first time were making the implied political commitment to reallocate scarce re-

Dr. Mosley served in Asia and Africa with the Ford Foundation as international health specialist. Currently Professor and Chairman of the Department of Population Dynamics, The John's Hopkins University School of Hygiene and Public Health, he is an acknowledged expert on international health and a frequent consultant to governments and health programs around the world.

sources from hospital-oriented medical systems toward community-oriented health strategies.

Among the driving forces behind the primary health care movement was the realization that health conditions in poor developing countries were not inextricably linked to the low levels of national income. For example, the populations of many relatively poor nations such as China, Sri Lanka, Costa Rica, Cuba, and of the State of Kerala in India, have levels of health and life expectancies that approach those seen in the affluent nations of the developed world. In those countries, the critical factor contributing to the better health that people enjoy is a commitment to equity in provision of basic health and other social services. In contrast to those nations, most developing countries have tended to invest the bulk of their health resources in sophisticated western-style hospitals which contribute relatively little to the health of the people. The urban bias of these institutions results in limited access to their services by the vast majority of the population who live in rural areas.

A recent assessment I carried out in a Middle Eastern country illustrates this situation. This country had developed a sophisticated medical system with a number of hospitals rivaling any institution in the western world. At present, however, because of unrestricted expansion of this western-style medical system, there is a surplus of hospital beds and hundreds of medical graduates are having difficulty finding employment. In spite of this, the government has still been committing 90% of its development funds in health to expanding the hospital bed capacity by 50% and to opening a second medical school. This is in a country where community health services are so inadequate that only 60% of the childbearing women receive any antenatal care and 40% of the deliveries are still done at home by unqualified midwives.

Priorities and response allocations

The primary health care movement involves first and foremost a redefinition of priorities toward the health needs of the community rather than to the desires of the medical profession. Following on this must come a reallocation of resources. This confronts us with a fundamental reality facing every health program, whether at the national level or in a mission hospital: the fact that rationing is inevitable.

For all practical purposes, only two alternatives exist. Health programs can either ration the numbers of people served or the numbers of conditions treated. The first alternative makes it possible to give a few individuals the "best" medical care that modern science can provide while the rest of the population receives little or nothing. Regrettably, this is the narrow orientation of many western-trained physicians who will demand that no expense is spared for sophisticated care of the few patients they personally attend, oblivious of the fact that they are indirectly depriving a far larger community of any health care whatsoever.

The alternative is to ration the number of diseases that are treated in order to assure that everyone at least has access to a basic level of essential services. This is the principle that underlies the PHC strategy. For example, a country could determine that it would postpone establishing an open heart surgery unit, which might meet the needs of a tiny (elite) fraction of the population, until an effective maternal and child health program is implemented assuring that every mother has antenatal and safe childbirth care, and every child is immunized.

Strategic Alternatives

For those countries or organizations that accept PHC in principle, there is still the unresolved issue of how to most effectively implement a program. Currently, most PHC strategies could be grouped into two broad categories; the institutional approach and the technological approach.

The Institutional Approach

The institutional approach basically seeks to graft elements of primary health care onto existing hospital and clinic-based medical systems with the goal of seeking to reach everyone in the community with a minimum range of basic services. This involves attempts to modify the existing health system by setting up some kind of an outreach program at the community level with a mechanism of referral to facilitate access to more complex care when needed. In terms of implementation, the typical approach is to develop a cadre of low-level community health workers. Coupled with this will usually be efforts to mobilize the community leaders to support the system through the establishment of village health committees.

A recent analysis of more than 50 such primary health care programs found most having serious operational problems. The difficulty was that while the medical institutions could construct facilities and train workers, they were generally unable to adequately support the system with logistics, medication, communication and supervision. Moreover, many of these projects were unable to maintain community participation and rarely did they become self supporting. Over a period of time, many projects, in order to maintain financial viability, would have the community health workers drop all the preventive services and become low-level, curative practitioners on a fee-for-service basis.

We must recognize this institutional approach has some inherent weaknesses. First, most programs typically maintain the traditional top-down approach of the centrally-managed medical institution. There is a failure to grasp the intrinsic differences between operating an extension program and building a decentralized community-based health program. Furthermore, most administrations have no training and experience with supporting highly decentralized, far-flung activities. Second, and linked to the first, the extension programs typically take no account of the traditional caring systems for managing diseases and disabilities that have had a long and self-sustaining existence in the community; rather, they seek to impose in its entirety all the drugs and therapies of western medicine. Such an approach is not only highly inefficient but may prove relatively ineffective because of the failure of the community to accept many of the treatments and preventative measures offered.

Finally, one reason that many of these institutional-based approaches flounder is because they begin with a "blueprint" approach; that is, with an a priori commitment to a certain type of organizational structure and health management system. They then devote almost all of their attention to maintaining the financial viability of the predetermined operation. What is needed is a more flexible "learning process" approach that assesses the health conditions in the community and the pre-existing health care systems, and works with the community leaders in their social context to define the best methods for improving the situation.

The Technological Approach

The technological approach can be epitomized by the strategy of "selective primary health care" (SPHC). SPHC is currently being promoted by agencies such as UNICEF and USAID as a programmatic alternative to implementing a comprehensive primary health care program. This strategy is based on the selection of a limited number of health interventions based on the identification of high priority health problems which have a high feasibility of being effectively controlled by existing technologies. Currently the two major interventions being promoted worldwide are immunizations and oral rehydration therapy for diarrhea. Increasingly, attention is being given to acute respiratory diseases and to nutrition (especially vitamin A deficiency).

In essence, SPHC is technology-driven, with maximum effort given to making the selected interventions widely available to entire populations. In contrast to the institutional approach, this technological approach virtually bypasses the entire health system. These interventions are largely built on such techniques as mass communication, public mobilization, and social marketing programs. Organizationally, SPHC may at times also operate like a vertical health program, built largely around low-level community health workers.

Selective primary health care has been criticized on numerous counts.

1. The very method of setting priorities on the basis of specific diseases automatically eliminates programmatic strategies which may protect against multiple diseases and disabilities simultaneously such as water and sanitation programs, the promotion of personal hygiene, antenatal and childbirth care, and family planning.

2. The proponents of the strategy grossly overestimate the lifesaving benefits of a specific intervention because they fail to take into account the interaction of multiple infections coupled with malnutrition that simultaneously lead to death among children growing up in impoverished communities.

3. There is the failure to appreciate the fact that these technical interventions, such as oral rehydration, may not be accepted or effectively used by people in traditional societies.

Two principles embedded in this selective primary health care strategy are important to recognize. The first is that the priorities for health interventions should be based on the health needs in the community. Second, an effective program must be population-based; that is, efforts must be made to reach every individual with the service if a health benefit is to be expected. The weakness of the selective primary health care strategy as presently being implemented is that too much is being promised by the application of a few interventions through mass campaign approaches, and inadequate attention is being given to building local capacity for self-sustaining health institutions.

Concepts in Community Health Care

To develop a primary health care program that is truly person-oriented as well as community-based, we need to appreciate exactly who is primarily involved in the production of healthy families and communities as well as to enunciate the critical values embedded in the primary health care philosophy. We must recognize that individuals and families in general, and mothers in particular, are truly the "producers" of health. This turns on its head our more traditional view of physicians as the "providers" and patients as the "consumers" of medical services. For example, in the case of child survival, the critical health provider is the mother. Her ability to produce healthy offspring will be facilitated or constrained by the beliefs and knowledge she has about disease causation, and by the skills, power, and resources she has to effectively act on that knowledge.

If we accept this perspective, then it becomes clear that the primary role of a health system should be to enhance the capacity of mothers and families to produce health among all their offspring and members. This will be achieved primarily by enhancing their understanding of disease causation, by adding to the skills and, where necessary, by providing resources and facilities for selected technical interventions which would be effectively available to everyone. In essence this implies that the orientation of a health system should be active and population-based, concerned with preserving and maintaining health rather than following the usual passive, institution-based model concerned with treating diseases.

In this conceptualization, a health program must go beyond clinical practice, and look to transforming the social and economic institutions in the community. A parallel can be drawn from the field of agriculture. We have no difficulty in looking upon individual families as the primary producers of agricultural products rather than the consumers of agricultural inputs. Thus it becomes obvious that the role of an agricultural program is not simply to disseminate crop-enhancing technologies such as insecticides and fertilizers, but also to promote the skills of the producers, reorganize social institutions, and develop infrastructures such as irrigation systems, markets, and even determine the prices of commodities in order to improve agricultural productivity.

This "systems" approach to agricultural development must have its parallel in health development. Too often health programs are narrowly conceived by most health professionals as consisting only of those medical facilities and services controlled by doctors. In fact, however, health professionals must become aware of all the social and economic barriers to good health in the community and then work hand-in-hand with the people to find the solutions to overcome them. For large areas of the developing world, one of the greatest constraints to better family health, especially for mothers and children, is the degraded status of women. Unless this and other unjust social institutions are addressed by health programs, little progress can be expected.

Basic Principles

If we accept individuals and families as the primary producers of health, and physicians and health professionals as only facilitators in the process, this means that we, as health professionals, must have a wholly new set of values and standards to guide our thinking and our actions. The usual values associated with Western medical practice are wholly inadequate to the task. It is at this point of conflict between values that the primary health care revolution is truly occurring.

A comparison between the traditional values implicit in Western medical practice and the new set of standards and principles that are essential to effective primary health care programs can be seen in the table on the facing page.

Two basic premises should be emphasized. First, the ultimate performance of any health care program is only measurable in terms of improved health among the people. This looking beyond ourselves contrasts with what I have seen in medical programs around the world. Typically, I am proudly shown new buildings or sophisticated equipment, or told about advanced surgical procedures being performed, or presented with pages of service statistics. Only exceptionally have I found institutions that could give me an accurate picture of the actual health conditions in the community, much less objective indicators of the progress that had been made to improve the situation. Some examples of these are given in this volume.

Western Medicine and Primary Health Care

ITEM	WESTERN MEDICINE	PRIMARY HEALTH CARE
REFERENCE POINT FOR JUDGING EXCELLENCE:	Medical standard defined by profession	Level of health/welfare as defined by community
INDICATORS OF HIGH QUALITY PERFORMANCE:	Higher education of specialists; sophistication of facilities	Self-reliance of people; coverage of population
BASIS FOR SETTING PRIORITIES:	New advances in western medicine	Local needs
EDUCATIONAL STRATEGY:	Prolonged; theoretical; biologically focused, reductionist	Brief, practical; behaviorally focused, integrative
ORIENTATION OF PRACTITIONER:	Closed, defensive, authoritative	Open, self-critical listening
COMMUNICATION TYPE:	Top-down	Two-way
EXPECTED RESPONSE:	Unquestioning obedience	Understanding cooperation
PROGRAM STRATEGY:	Institution-based technology-oriented; What to do?	Community-based; process-oriented; How to do?
PROGRAM EVALUATION:	Services performed by practitioners	Results produced in the community
RELATIONSHIP TO INDIGENOUS PRACTITIONERS:	Competitive, undermining credibility; limit their role; reduce their skills	Supportive partnership, expand their role; enhance their skills
IMPACT ON INDIVIDUALS AND THE COMMUNITY:	Weaken initiative; produce dependency	Strengthen initiative; produce autonomy

The second premise is no less important. Community-based primary health care programs must be as much concerned about the process of improving health among people as they are about the outcome. Health in a family or a community is measured not only by the improvements in physical or biological parameters but also by the degree to which they have grown in initiative, autonomy and self-reliance. If this becomes the ultimate goal in the planning, development and implementation of health programs, then the root cause of failure of so many efforts — lack of community involvement and support — is avoided. Health professionals will find that rather than struggling to enlist the community to support their externally conceived action plans, they will be supporting the community as it develops a wholeness in every dimension — physically, socially, economically and spiritually.

Questions for Reflection

1. What do you think may have been some of the driving forces behind the development of the primary health care movement?

2. Contrast the priorities of the health needs of communities in your country with the usual priorities of the medical profession.

3. What are some of the advantages and disadvantages of the institutional approach discussed in this chapter? Of the technological approach?

4. How do you respond to the statement that "families, and mothers in particular, are the producers of health"? Have you been accustomed to thinking of medical professionals as producers of health? Why or why not?

5. What are some of the political, socio-economic, and spiritual barriers to good health in your community?

6. What reasonable steps could medical institutions take to get a more accurate picture of the actual health conditions in the communities they serve?

5

Community-Based Health Development

Roy Shaffer, M.D., M.P.H.

Throughout history, people have intuitively believed that "prevention is better than cure" and that individual health is closely interrelated with community health. The Old Testament contains numerous references to the reciprocal responsibilities binding the Israelite people to each other and to their God in community health in its broadest sense.

This chapter attempts to show: 1) the traditional cure-dominated medical model of health is *inadequate* to address current health problems, 2) local communities could shoulder significantly more *responsibility* for their own health care, and 3) a better *balance* is needed between those health activities which are institution-based (I-B) and those that are community-based (C-B). These three issues will help to determine the extent to which there will be some improvement in health for all by the year 2,000.

Community Health in Historical Context

As early as 1850, a sanitary commission report in Massachusetts emphasized the importance of community and personal responsibility for improving health. This personal and community emphasis had little support for two reasons. First, the rapid development of municipal waterworks was dramatically reducing the prevalence of water-related diseases and thereby decreasing the pressure on community health promotional services. This "Era of Public Health" and its focus on pipes (water and waste) and regulations (hygiene and contagion) generated tremendous improvement of health of communities.

The son of missionary parents, Dr. Shaffer completed his medical training in the U.S. and then returned to East Africa where he served as a District Medical Officer. One of the original Flying Doctors of East Africa, he helped to develop and promote the basic principles of community-based health care throughout the region. He is currently the health development specialist for MAP International in East Africa.

Second, at the turn of the century, breakthroughs in bacteriology and immunization followed by new forms of chemotherapy resulted in an emphasis on "the men in white coats." There ensued both a popular and professional fixation on institution-centered health care which offered a "pill for every problem" or a "needle for every need." It raised the expectation that medicine could solve every health problem.

Following World War II, a greater emphasis was placed upon social perspectives of health. The term "Community Health" emerged as a label for what the World Health Organization (WHO) now considers the "eight essential elements of Primary Health Care." Although the perspective had become more community-oriented, the mode was still authoritarian and institution-based. This was true both in the West and the Third World. Meanwhile, the seriousness of problems was increasing faster than society's capacity to solve them.

The Advent of Primary Health Care

In the early 1970s, health care in the Third World was beset by many problems:

- Most countries lacked clean water, sanitation systems and enforceable health regulations.

- Society possessed neither the unity nor the resources to develop community services at the local level.

- Both villagers and health workers were more comfortable with a cure-centered system than one emphasizing disease prevention. To them, the former was more tangible, more immediate, easier to implement and seemingly more humanitarian and effective.

- Burgeoning populations were swamping and bankrupting the cure-centered system which these young governments were trying to administer and finance.

In the Third World, the health care system is based primarily on the *health center*. Of the illnesses treated there, at least half are avoidable. Yet despite decades of health education, people with these illnesses continue to appear, get treatment, go back to the same situation and reappear again and again. The *same* child with the *same* type ascaris infestation sees the *same* clinician, is given the *same* piperazine cure and goes back to the *same* unhygienic environment to be re-infested with the *same* problem — again and again.

In this situation, the health center becomes mainly a "recycling center," recycling illness that people could and should have prevented or treated themselves right in their own neighborhood.

At a WHO-UNICEF conference at Alma Ata (Soviet Union) in 1978, many of the world's nations adopted primary health care (PHC) as a major strategy for improving the quality and quantity of health care service. PHC was not presented as a new technology but rather as a shift of emphasis from institutions to the community. PHC was not to replace clinical care but rather proposed to broaden the spectrum of ways through which health problems would be addressed outside of health facilities. This implied a major adjustment of priorities on the part of the medical establishment.

The Alma Ata conference declaration proposed a health care system (PHC) that would be accessible, affordable and participatory. Although long on adjectives, the declaration was short on nouns and verbs specifying exactly *who* was going to do *what*. There was little discussion of *peoples' responsibility* for improving their own health or the critical importance of *communication skills* in promoting change. Discussions among health workers also reflected widespread uncertainty and ambiguity regarding the practical implications and interpretation of the title word "primary."

Community-Based Health Care (C-BHC)

In 1979, this author and others in East Africa posited community-based health care (C-BHC) as that part of primary health care which happens in the local community beyond the reach of curative services. C-BHC comprises those activities that local neighborhoods carry out by themselves to improve their own health apart from what health care institutions do for them. While C-BHC may be facilitated by outsiders, it should not be directed by outsiders. That would be a contradiction. For example, the community health worker should be more closely affiliated to her/his neighborhood leadership than to the outside project implementors. Unfortunately, the opposite usually happens.

C-BHC neither arises *de nouveau* nor exists in a vacuum. Any and all community health care includes a mixture of different activities launched from a variety of bases. Some care activities are institution-based and others are community-based. The two types are different but complementary. Tshimika's case study from Zaire in this volume suggests that when these two dimensions work together, health in a community improves.

The label "community-based" applies accurately only to those activities that are initiated and implemented primarily by the local neighborhood itself. People draw on their *own* initiative and their *own* resources, and carry on their *own* responsibilities. That is the meaning of "ownership." By this definition, the popular mobile clinic operation is only partially community-based. The vehicle, vaccines, cold chain and medical expertise are all institution-based.

Community-based health care concerns mainly that enhancement of health which occurs when motivated people *collectively* change their habits, improve their home conditions and become more self-reliant. It is a matter of acculturation and neighborhood norms. When people in a neighborhood regularly wash their hands after using the latrine or before eating, this will do more for community health than the existence of a "disease post," otherwise known as a dispensary. In C-BHC, the development of *people* is much more important than the creation of programs or facilities.

Facilitating Community-Based Health Care

An institution can only facilitate a community's initiatives aimed at producing their own C-BHC programs. This process of promoting or facilitating community- based health includes several dimensions:

● Transferring relevant *knowledge* in appropriate and effective ways.

● Motivating better *attitudes* toward self and health.

● Encouraging the adoption of better *habits*.

Several examples will illustrate. A mother's realization that eating green, leafy vegetables will restore normal color to an anemic child exemplifies the acquisition of knowledge. A couple's decision to request information regarding child-spacing often reflects an attitudinal change. Regular, family hand washing may indicate a change of habit or behavior.

These changes in knowledge, attitudes and habits are closely related. Of the three, attitudinal changes are probably the most crucial because they affect the community's sense of self-awareness, self-worth, self-confidence and therefore its ability to become self-reliant. Self-reliance is the essence of being "community-based."

Many health care professionals who promote community-based programs overlook the issue of attitudes. Instead, they emphasize the transfer of knowledge (the life-cycle of parasites, the composition of food groups, etc.) or focus on activities designed to produce visible results such as mass vaccination statistics and attendance at maternal-child clinics. These are good and certainly appropriate. However, they fail to get to the heart of the matter which is people's attitudes towards themselves, the world and change.

The most important objective for outside facilitators of community-based health care must be the evolution of self-awareness, self-worth, self-confidence and therefore self-reliance on the part of individuals and neighborhoods. This requires new communication skills and training practices that are generally not part of health education programs in the Third World.

The Community

Community development begins in a local neighborhood which is small enough that people:

● *Know* each other by name.

● *Feel* a sense of unity and trust and care for each other.

● *Share* responsibility for the health of the neighborhood.

In this kind of community, everyone feels themselves to be a health worker. Leaders and followers share a sense of reciprocal responsibility to each other. Neighbors care for each other's needs.

These responsibilities are woven together like the strands in a basket. Think of the vertical strands as the leadership roles within a community. Imagine the continuous circular strands to be the roles of the followers. The weaving together of strands running in opposite directions is what creates the basket. Similarly, community development is the product of the weaving together of two different types of responsibilities, those of community leaders and those of ordinary people in the community. There is no substitute for such reciprocal responsibilities. A basket cannot be held together by glue as a substitute for weaving. Likewise, community-based development cannot be glued together by outside money or resources.

The Evolution of Community-based Health Care

Health development programs which are community-based have tended to evolve according to a general pattern:

1. **Community awareness** - Progressive communities are driven or coaxed by outsiders into the realization that they are primarily responsible for their own health. They then commit themselves corporately and publicly to an initiative designed to change habits, improve conditions and promote self-reliance.

2. **Coordinating group** - An existing committee or its traditional equivalent might be assigned responsibility for initiating action somewhat along this line:

- Initiate public discussion of local problems, identifying and prioritizing those that are solvable by the community.

- Secure agreement on one change that will be introduced first. Determine the means through which it will be addressed.

- Identify resource people to bring skills in evaluation, communication, management and technical information regarding these problems.

- Promote creative community discussion of community-based information system to monitor progress toward the change objective.

- Elicit a commitment by individuals and the community to actively implement the change in specified ways on a specified schedule.

3. **Corporate action** - The acid-test of community-based development is whether or not the community implements the plans that it has made. Where there is no corporate action, there can be no community-based development.

4. **Community health workers (CHWs)** - The presence of CHWs does not make programs community-based. CHWs can only facilitate the process. If they are part of C-BHC, their roles must be clearly defined and

candidates carefully screened and appropriately trained. CHWs have successfully provided institution-based services in the community but have done less well in serving as catalysts of local initiatives.

5. **Supervision** - The leadership group must then continuously monitor everyone's contribution and evaluate the progress being made. Objective evidence of progress (i.e. disappearance of scabies, etc.) enhances the community's sense of self-worth, self-confidence and therefore self-reliance.

The Christian Perspective

What are the implications of community-based health care for Christian health workers? They should be the most sensitive of all to the relatively greater importance in development of people over things or programs. In the Christian perspective, "personal development" includes a dimension which is hardly considered by the secular world. This is the spiritual dimension which comes with the conversion experience.

This new life in Christ can and should revolutionize the new believer's attitude to his/her health and the environment that God has created. People who are thus transformed should be at the cutting edge of community health development. They will be busy, both *doing* and *being* like God in a lovingly careful life (see I John 3:16-18). This reflects the fact that community development is indeed an "inside" job. Christians with this kind of motivation should be the least dependent upon the motivations, initiatives and resources of outsiders. This applies to individuals and congregations.

Donor agencies handling Christian, sacrificially-given funds should try to allocate those funds to "Christ-Based Health Care" initiatives. They should ponder the ethics of funding a neighborhood from which they have not been able to elicit any community-based initiative, resources or responsibilities.

Conclusion

Communities *can* be successfully motivated to improve their habits and conditions. Christians, with their yet-deeper spiritual motivations can enable the Church to lead the way toward better community health. But these are conditional upon three fundamental changes in belief:

- The medical establishment has to believe more in *people*.
- People have to believe more in *themselves*.
- Both have to believe more in the *feasibility* and *necessity* of preventing most illnesses by changing the local community's own habits and conditions.

It is a matter of balance.

Questions for Reflection

1. The author states that throughout history, people have intuitively believed that prevention is better than cure. Do you agree? Can you give examples to illustrate this?

2. What have been some of the major problems in providing health care in the Third World? What would be some "do-able" steps in solving these problems?

3. Discuss the interrelatedness of the three dimensions in facilitating community-based health: gaining knowledge, motivating attitudes, and adopting better habits. Is one more important than the other? Why or why not?

4. Name several fundamental changes in belief that usually need to occur to lead the way toward better community health.

5. Have you ever felt responsible for the health of the members in your immediate community? What factors have influenced your own attitudes in this regard?

6

Vanga: Health, the Church and the Government

Daniel E. Fountain, M.D.

One of the many legacies that western civilization brought to the Third World is the compartmentalization of life and responsibilities. Medical care is the responsibility of doctors, nurses and hospitals. Evangelism and church growth are the responsibility of evangelists and pastors. Administration, law and order are the responsibility of government. Public health — preventative medicine — has long been considered part of the government's domain. Overlap between the domains of the church and the government has been minimal. The cooperation between the two has been limited. In addition, ordinary people have played a very small role in the delivery of health care services.

The theme of this chapter is that the church can play an important role in overcoming this compartmentalization between the church and the state. By involving the people in a basic health program, the church can change a "medical service" into a "health ministry." By cooperating effectively and influentially with government health leaders, the church can help reorient national health policies toward community-based and integrated health care and development. The church-based community health program at Vanga in the Republic of Zaire is an example of what can be done in bringing change into both government and church health policies.

The Vanga Health Program

The Vanga Evangelical Hospital served as a small rural, general hospital for forty years during the colonial regime in what was then the Belgian Congo. The hospital had a very active curative program with

Dr. Fountain served for more than twenty five years as a medical missionary in Zaire with the American Baptist Foreign Mission Society. His pioneering work in community health development has been a model for other mission hospitals and the Ministry of Health in Zaire. Dr. Fountain is now part of MAP International's training staff in Brunswick, Georgia.

emphasis on general surgery. This medical program gained the confidence of the people in modern medical care. The program was closely related to the church in both evangelism and church growth, with the medical staff participating in village evangelism and in the strengthening of local church congregations.

In 1961, the medical service at Vanga underwent a basic change in orientation from a strictly medical program to an integrated health program. Two compelling factors brought about this change.

First, in 1960 Belgium granted Zaire its independence and the well-developed colonial medical service soon almost ceased to function. As a result, the church health services had to play a crucial role in the provision of health care for the people. The Vanga Hospital became the only hospital for a population of a quarter of a million people. But a single general hospital with only two physicians could never provide adequate health care for such a large population.

Second, a very high percentage of patients coming to the hospital were suffering from preventable diseases. It was evident that many of the same patients were returning again and again with the same illnesses. In spite of the curative care given, no evident improvement occurred in the health of the people.

For example, a mother brought her three-year old boy to the hospital suffering from weight loss, abdominal pain and distension and vomiting. The boy had ascaris eggs in his stools. Six hours after receiving a worm treatment, the boy developed signs of intestinal obstruction. In spite of insufficient skills in pediatric surgery and anesthesia, we performed a laparotomy and removed 492 ascaris worms from the small intestine. The boy recovered quickly and went home after ten days, a triumph of surgery and prayer. But four months later, his mother brought him again to the hospital, malnourished, with another heavy burden of ascaris. What had we really accomplished?

As our orientation toward community health care began to develop, we established four goals:

1. To make primary health care services available to the entire population of 250,000 persons.

2. To involve the people themselves in efforts to improve their own health, transferring to them as much responsibility as possible for planning health activities and applying measures to improve health.

3. To work through the local church in our community health program, thus strengthening and extending the ministry and influence of the church.

4. To show to the government effective ways of improving the health of the people.

Structure and Organization

In order to implement the change in orientation from a "medical" to a "health" ministry, and from an "institutional" to a "community" program, several measures were adopted at the hospital level. This was necessary to permit the hospital to serve as the base for the community health program.

1. **Training of personnel.** A community health program requires personnel trained in the principles and application of primary health care and community development. In 1962, we opened a school for training paramedical community health personnel, and slowly it began to meet the need for primary health care personnel. We gave short courses to existing paramedical personnel to help them become able to function in primary and community health programs. We trained auxiliary personnel to assist the paramedical staff in health centers and in the communities and to work in maternities and in small rural laboratories. This, of course, made it necessary for us doctors to learn how to teach and to be willing to invest the time necessary to do it well. We still have much to learn.

2. **Reorganization of the hospital.** Good organization is necessary for effective functioning. The Vanga Hospital was poorly organized and much time and effort were required of the professional staff to make the hospital function satisfactorily. With better management policies and the training of local staff in administration, our professional staff had more time available for teaching, organizing and working on the community level.

3. **The hospital as example.** As planning for our community health program began, a consultation was held with our local church leaders. During the discussion, our local pastor asked how we thought we could involve people in the villages in adopting habits of cleanliness and hygiene when our hospital itself was so filthy and unhygienic. What his question lacked in tact was more than made up for in veracity. A year was set aside to improve the hospital facilities, inside and out, in order to serve better as a model of health behavior.

4. **Delegation of responsibilities.** Our professional staff required much time to meet the urgent curative needs of patients. Yet many of the services required were relatively simple. So we began training mature members of our paramedical staff to handle many of the acute and less-complicated medical and surgical problems such as obstructed deliveries, simple hernia repairs, uncomplicated fractures and more complex problems of diagnosis and medical treatment.

By effective training and delegation of responsibilities to trained paramedical colleagues, followed by regular supervision, the professional staff was able to devote less time to the urgent and more to the important. The extra time required for this training and delegation proved to be a very efficient long-term investment of time and effort.

Central Themes

Involvement of the Church and the Population in Health

From the very beginning, we envisaged the community health program as a church-based program. We had several reasons for this.

- The church exists in almost all villages and is therefore a community structure.

- The church has considerable influence in village affairs and, with some training and motivation of its leaders, can be a permanent and continuing influence in matters relating to health and development.

- Many of the problems affecting health are social and spiritual. These include problems of integrity, trust, responsibility and a worldview of passive acceptance of difficulties including disease and death.

- The most effective approach is the application of God's Word to these problems, and the local church is the obvious structure for teaching and promoting application of God's Word.

The church-based community health program at Vanga began in 1967 with a series of weekend seminars at church centers. These consisted of group dialogues with village pastors, chiefs and elders. During these discussions we discovered the wealth of insight in the Bible concerning human relations and how social and spiritual order is related to health. We likewise discovered ways to use traditional concepts in order to explain new ideas. Rather than trying to refute traditional beliefs, which would in effect be refuting the people who hold these beliefs, the use of some of these beliefs with reinterpretations proved effective in transmitting new ideas. For example, the traditional concept of the curse comes from the belief that one person can cause another person to become ill. The "transmission" is invisible and usually through magical means. This belief resembles in some ways the science of contagion according to which disease transmission, although by physical and measurable means, is indeed often invisible.

Acceptance and application of these ideas in terms of changed behavior came slowly, but progressively, pastors and Christian elders helped promote the new ideas of health and development.

The initial programs in community health were related to improving village sanitation and maternal and child health. Problems of nutrition, family planning, endemic disease control, agricultural production and the protection of the environment came later. From the very beginning, each village was encouraged to create a "development committee" of responsible leaders to take charge of the development efforts in the village. We called these committees "development" committees rather than health committees because of the strong relationship between health and all aspects of develop-ment.

Relationships with the Government Health Service

From its earliest days, the Vanga hospital has been accredited by the National Health Ministry as a church-based private hospital. From the beginning, contacts have been frequent between the leaders of the Vanga health program and the Ministry of Health. Regular reports are sent, and correspondence is frequent. All programs conform to the norms established by the Health Ministry. No changes or new initiatives are made without permission of the Ministry.

However, as the village sanitation program began to grow, considerable opposition came from the local government health officers. These officers were responsible for the inspection of sanitary installations in the villages, and they feared an undermining of their authority. They likewise obtained less revenues for fines levied on those lacking satisfactory sanitary installations. Because of their complaints, the Regional Doctor wrote to us in 1970 forbidding us to continue our community health activities. Our role, he said, was limited strictly to curative medicine. "Public health" was the domain of the government. But after a personal visit to the national Health Minister, this situation was resolved and the Minister not only allowed but actually encouraged us to continue.

On the other hand, the government administrative leaders on the local and regional levels were delighted with the changes taking place in the health conditions of the people. They perceived and appreciated the value of the changes that were occurring. They now recognize the value of the village development committees and in many cases actively encourage their activities.

In 1975 the Minister of Health, formerly a professor of public health at the National University of Zaire, invited us to explain the Vanga community health program to the annual meeting of the Regional Doctors from all over Zaire. During the discussion that followed, the Minister of Health made it clear that from that time forward all competition between government and private health services was finished. Not only would there be cooperation; there would also be a sharing of responsibilities for all aspects of the health care of the people.

Two months later several church health leaders participated in a planning session convened by the Minister of Health to plan the structure and functioning of what became known as a "Rural Health Zone." According to the plan, each functioning hospital, regardless of affiliation, would be responsible for the technical organization and supervision of all of the health activities in its catchment areas. Following this workshop, the Vanga hospital was given the responsibilities for the organization and supervision of all government and church-related dispensaries and health centers in its zone of action. The Vanga Rural Health Zone became the second such zone in Zaire.

Although it has required almost ten years for this Rural Health Zone plan to be officially adopted and put into effect, the development of rural and now urban health zones has followed the guidelines drawn up in the original planning session. The experiences gained in the Vanga Rural Health Zone were instrumental in drawing up the original plan, and they have been very useful in planning and organizing many other government and church-related health zones in the country.

The Vanga community health program has influenced national health policy in other areas as well.

1. **Importance of Community Participation.** Community participation is a new departure in development activities in Zaire. Originally a politically sensitive issue, the example of constructive activity on the local level by village development committees in the Vanga Health Zone and subsequently in many others has encouraged the government to adopt this principle as part of national health policy. Official policies are likewise moving in this direction in other areas of development.

2. **Integration on the Village Level**. Several other ministries of the government have also become interested in community participation. Initially each ministry wanted to establish its own "agent" in each village. One agent would be responsible for health, one for hygiene, one for water improvement, another for environmental control and yet another for agricultural development. However, in various planning sessions, the example in our church programs of the integration that existed in the village development committees convinced the government that such "compartmentalization" would be ineffective. As a result, the village development committees continue their integrated activities, working together on all of the various development needs in their communities.

3. **Integration on the Health Zone Level**. The national Ministry of Health operates "vertical" programs within the ministry. The Expanded Program of Immunizations and separate programs for nutrition and for the control of diseases such as tuberculosis, African sleeping sickness and malaria each have their own programs and budgets. However, on the Health Zone level, our church-based health leaders made major efforts to coordinate the different activities and to integrate the various "vertical" programs into the Zone structure. As a result, the integration of these programs on the Zone level is now national health policy.

4. **Suppression of Fining as a Method of Motivation**. One of the holdovers from the colonial administration has been the strong emphasis on sanctions such as the levying of fines for bringing about behavior change. Although this method has never been effective, it continues to be used in various government programs. However, in community health programs, behavior change is brought about only through effective education. Sanctions such as fining generally have a negative effect.

The effectiveness of the church-based community health programs based on education and positive motivational factors has been evident to government leaders. Although the practice of levying fines continues to be used in some areas on a widespread scale, there is a growing tendency to limit this strictly to the most recalcitrant problems.

Lessons Learned

During the more than 25 years of involvement in the Vanga community health program, many lessons have been learned.

1. **People as resource**. People are the primary resource for development and the improvement of health.

2. **Integrated health**. Health is a way of life, a manner of living, with implications far beyond medicine, hygiene and curative health care.

3. **Obstacles to health and development**. The principle obstacles to health and development are social, moral and spiritual. The primary resources for overcoming these obstacles are God's Word and the Spirit of Jesus Christ working in the community of God's people.

4. **The church in development**. The church is ideally suited for effective work in health and development. With a solid moral and spiritual foundation, the wealth of insight from God's Word, its emphasis on positive relationships and its village-based structure, the church can bring about basic changes in beliefs, attitudes and behavior.

5. **Community health care**. An important distinction exists between primary health care and community health care. Primary health care consists of those activities done by the health services for and with the population to improve the health of the people. Community health care consists of all activities initiated and carried on by the community to improve the health of the people. Primary health care and community health care are complementary. But the health services must never diminish or supplant local community initiatives. On the contrary, all health interventions should be done in such a way as to motivate and strengthen community initiative.

6. **Cultural sensitivity**. Health professionals who wish to work effectively in community health must be able to understand the cultural beliefs and values of the people with whom they work. They likewise must be fluent in their language and be able to communicate with them in culturally effective ways.

7. **Strengthening national policy**. The church can play a positive role in affecting national health policy. This requires adequate communication, regular reports, conformity to official policy and standards as well as frequent personal contacts with health care administrators. Through diplomacy and with positive examples developed through experience, an

effective church-based health program can be instrumental in promoting changes in local and even national health programs. God's Word can be a light even for the making of health policy. His people can likewise be a light to show the way to integrated health.

Questions for Reflection

1. What are some of the dangers of compartmentalizing responsibilities and roles in the provision of health care?

2. In this case study, what role has the church assumed in providing health care to people in the region? What impact has this role had on the ministry of the church?

3. What does this case study suggest about the relationship of church-sponsored, community-based development programs to governments?

4. How might the church motivate people to make behavioral changes that would lead to improved health?

5. This case study described how a Christian health development program helped to shape national policy. How could your church affect the health policy in your country or community?

7

Case Study: Health Development in the Rural United States

Peter A. Boelens, M.D.

What a shock to return to the United States after six years of medical mission work in Korea during the turbulent 1960s. The country to which I returned had changed in my absence. My homeland wore a different face and had a different heartbeat. During subsequent training at the University of Minnesota, my fellow students and faculty constantly reminded me that Christianity was irrelevant to the needs of American society.

"Christians are mainly interested in themselves and their children rather than the poor people in the slums," they said. "You have no concern for the poor at your own doorstep." Although I had just spent several years caring for the poor overseas, these comments made me feel that I was ignoring the needs of hurting people in my own country.

Such accusations motivated my wife and me to ask God for clear direction in our lives. He soon made it evident that we were to begin a mission work within the U.S. This chapter describes how this decision was translated into a community health development program in the southern United States.

Rural Mississippi

Having attended medical school and completed an internship in Chicago, I expected to launch a ministry in a large northern, urban ghetto area. The Lord, however, had other ideas. After extensive investigation, we discovered that the rural South, particularly the Mississippi Delta, was both an area of extreme need, and a place where we as Christians could have a definite impact.

After serving as a missionary physician in Korea for six years, Dr. Boelens returned home to the U.S. where he initiated a community health development program in Cary, Mississippi. He is currently the Executive Director of The Luke Society, an organization of medical and dental professionals dedicated to world missions.

The Delta extends from Memphis, Tennessee to Vicksburg, Mississippi. This area contains some of the richest farm land in the nation, but it is also a region with third-world-type poverty. The economy of the area was based on cotton, soybeans, rice, and catfish. Large landowners who farmed between 1,000 and 10,000 acres dominated the area economically and politically. The region had little industry.

A few rich plantation owners, a small middle class, and a large number of poor made up the social structure. The poor were mainly black farm laborers who had been replaced by mechanization. One mechanical cotton picker displaced more than 100 farm laborers. With few jobs available locally, many people emigrated to northern cities in search of employment.

The 1970 census revealed the poverty in Sharkey county, the location of our Mississippi ministry. According to government statistics, 45 percent of the families in the county fell below the poverty line. Of these families, the median annual income was $1,907.00. Health statistics echoed the dismal situation. The 1968-1970 average infant mortality rate was 49.2 deaths per thousand live births, three times higher than the national average.

The Beginning

Our goal was to provide access to health care and to reduce the high infant mortality rate in the area. To accomplish this, we opened a Christian community health clinic in the delta town of Cary. From the beginning, our philosophy was not to meet all of the area's health care needs but rather to function as a catalyst for change. This meant collaborating with other agencies and individuals in the state.

Our clinic required subsidies since patients otherwise unable to afford health care were charged a reduced fee. The amount of this fee depended on the size of the household and the family income. A high percentage of our patients had no insurance, nor did they qualify for Medicaid (government health insurance for the poor). They were the working poor who had nowhere else to turn for health care.

Total Person Health Care

As Christians, we wanted to offer total person health care. The program's curative aspects opened doors and gave credence to our health education and spiritual ministries. Being funded primarily by Christians also gave us the flexibility to address people's needs without being stymied by government bureaucracy or the constraints of funding agencies.

We started classes for mothers on how to take care of themselves during pregnancy and their infants after delivery. This has been extremely successful, given the high incidence of environmental retardation in the area. Through our parenting and infant stimulation classes, people learned how to maximize the intellectual development of their children. Studies have shown that environment can make as much as a twenty-point difference in IQ.

The lack of transportation emerged as a glaring need early in the program. Sick people could not easily get to the clinic, so they waited until the very last moment before seeking health care. The consequences to health were often serious. Others could not participate in preventive health care programs or attend health education classes. To alleviate this problem, we established a system to transport patients from the remote corners of the county to the clinic.

The problems seen in the clinic were often just the tip of the iceberg. An outreach program, we decided, could investigate these needs in greater depth. An example of the problem was a child who came to the clinic with severe heat rash and secondary infection. Sores covered the child from head to foot. The mother explained that the family lived in a trailer without air conditioning or water. The public health nurse investigated and found that the 60-home community in which this family lived had only a sporadic water supply since the community well had run dry following an extremely hot summer. The public health department was mobilized to provide potable water to the residents. They sought a grant from the Federal Home Administration to link the community to the city water system. Although emergency funds were available, they would not be released for another six months.

An exciting thing happened in the midst of a seemingly hopeless situation. Outside volunteers joined with community members to install a new water system for approximately one-quarter of the commercial cost. At the conclusion of the laborious project, a grateful community honored the volunteers with a picnic to show appreciation for the help they had received.

We witnessed many other examples of how volunteers performed repairs on substandard houses or assisted in the construction of new homes for working families.

Training

In order to provide better care for residents of the delta, I became maternal child health care director for the county health department. In this capacity, I was able to organize a system for the care of mothers, infants and children. Treatment was initiated in the county health department. They then channeled patients to appropriate health facilities in a nearby town, and from there the patients were referred as necessary to the closest medical center. In addition, through our efforts the University and State Board of Health established a Children and Youth Project in nearby Vicksburg, which offered pediatric, dental, hearing, speech and psychological services. This facility became the hub of referral for outlying counties.

It soon became apparent that better trained primary health care workers were needed in many of the county health departments if people without insurance were to have access to quality health care. On this basis, we established a pediatric nurse associate program at the University of Mississippi School of Nursing. Initially federally funded, the state of Mississippi eventually financed the program. This program trained public health nurses from surrounding counties to care for poor children in their own communities. Although this action resulted in superb health care for poor families, cutbacks in state funding ultimately forced the cancellation of the program.

Examinations in the clinic constantly revealed youngsters classified as "failures to thrive" — malnourished, underweight and underheight. Some of these children were products of maternal neglect while others came from homes where mothers lacked sufficient funds to purchase infant formulas. In spite of an extensive nutrition education program, many mothers were reluctant to breast-feed the children. To address the problem of malnutrition, Cary Christian Health Center provided the research data necessary for the State Board of Health to establish the first WIC (Women, Infant, and Children) food program in the state. This aid made a noticeable difference.

After the introduction of the WIC program, the number of children diagnosed as "failures to thrive" decreased significantly. Those children who continued to suffer from this condition were usually victims of maternal neglect. This necessitated working closely with their mothers in conjunction with other state agencies.

Although our clinic maintained its independence, we coordinated our efforts and worked very closely with governmental agencies in the state. The federal government also provided assistance through the National Health Service Corps, from which our physicians and dentists were funded. However, once again, this program has been discontinued due to a cutback in funding.

Results

What has changed? The infant mortality rate plunged by over 50 percent from 50 to 22 deaths per 1,000 live births by 1972-1975. This marked reduction resulted from a multifaceted, integrated program which impacted on high risk mothers and their children. Mothers learned to better care for themselves and their infants.

The nurse-midwives in the charity hospital where most of the mothers in this program delivered noticed the difference. They reported that mothers coming from our program fared much better during labor and delivery than those not from the program. Our mothers were more attuned to what was happening. They also related to their infants in a more appropriate manner. This could also be seen in the clinics. At the beginning of this program, diarrhea leading to dehydration was a common problem.

After several years, it rarely became necessary to hospitalize a baby for this condition. The mothers had learned to give appropriate treatment.

Perhaps the most visible change in the community was the injection of hope into an apparently hopeless situation. Individuals have blossomed and assumed leadership roles in the community. The leader of the spiritual program, for example, was once a member of a small group Bible study initiated by our clinic. From his Bible teaching program, local churches have gained qualified teachers. Some have returned as summer volunteers at the Center, investing their lives in others. A definite health impact has been made, but it is the changed lives in Jesus Christ that really stand out and make a difference in the community.

Lessons Learned

A number of lessons have been learned through this community health program in the Mississippi Delta:

1. **Poverty on our doorstep.** It is very evident that the richest country in the world has pockets of third-world poverty in its midst. In these pockets of poverty, Christians are praying and crying for help. A pastor in Cary said, "We've been praying for a long, long time for God's help, and we look to Cary Christian Health Center as God's answer to our prayers." I wonder how many other needy Christians in the rural and urban areas of our country are raising similar petitions to the Lord?

2. **Bridging the gap.** In recent years, the United States has experienced some dramatic socio-economic shifts which have given us an "underclass" in our urban ghettos. We also see an ever-enlarging number of rural poor whose needs now surpass their urban counterparts. Most of us live in isolation from these poor and so we miss their cries for help. Even when we hear them, we still do not fully comprehend the magnitude of their problem.

At the end of his medical career, a physician friend became the public health officer in his home district. He confided that although he had practiced in the area for his entire professional life, he was amazed at the large number of poor in the district who lacked medical care.

We need bridges that connect the "haves" and the "have nots." Programs such as the Cary Christian Health Center serve as bridges into poor communities. Individuals can cross that bridge and become personally involved with the poor. As a result, the lives of the poor are enhanced and the individuals ministering have a mind and heart-expanding experience that redirects their thinking and priorities in life.

Since it was established, Cary has provided this kind of exposure for over four thousand volunteers who have come to help. We have seen young people change careers, retirees start new careers and others go into full-time ministry with the poor because of their contacts with the "have nots." They have experienced the fulfillment of bridging this gap in a meaningful way.

3. **Long-term commitment.** Poverty is a problem with deep and complex roots. There are no short-term solutions. Individuals and families need to move from hopelessness to hope by learning to take responsibility for their own lives and in the process learn to solve their own problems. For this to happen, they need friends who know them personally and will share the pilgrimage. This requires time and a long-term commitment.

This discipling process is impossible with a constant turnover in an organization's personnel. Relationships are established only to be broken. As a result, individuals being helped experience a sense of frustration and abandonment. Thankfully, the Cary Center's Christian staff have made long-term commitments, making it possible to invest in people.

Some of the present staff members are the result of this type of involvement. They are now investing their lives in others. This kind of return requires a minimum of five to ten years. It often takes this amount of time to disciple individuals and bring them to the point of maturity where they in turn are discipling others. It is this approach, however, which brings about lasting, long-term gains.

4. **Coordination.** Access to basic primary health care, like basic education for children, is usually considered a governmental responsibility. In order to address the complex problems of poverty in the delta, we coordinated our efforts with the existing health care system. We collaborated with other church and voluntary agencies. We worked within the infrastructure of the region, assisting the government in meeting its goals. In this process, the program has been able to interject a compassionate, caring and Christlike attitude. In doing this we not only function as salt in society, but also as a shining light.

5. **Catalysts for change.** The initial intent of the Luke Society in establishing a medical outreach in Cary was not to meet all the health care needs in Sharkey and Issaquena Counties but rather to assist existing agencies to meet the needs of the poor in a more effective manner. In order to accomplish this, we worked at the University Medical Center, University School of Nursing, Department of Health and the State Charity Hospital in addition to our ministry at Cary.

The clinic program at Cary Christian Health Center became the base from which we established a broad range of creative programs for the poor. Many of these programs were then incorporated into the programs of existing state agencies. The Cary Health Center also served as an agency with whom the state could contract in order to initiate new programs or expand existing programs.

One example of this is a nurse practitioner educational program we initiated at the University School of Nursing. The majority of students were public health nurses under scholarship from the State Board of Health. These nurses returned to their health departments and became points of entry for many poor children into the health care system.

Another example is a regional system for newborn care established in conjunction with the Charity Hospital, State Board of Health and University Medical Center. Within this system, all babies delivered were visited at home within the first week of life. High risk environmental situations were identified and appropriate preventive measures taken.

These and many other programs were established because we avoided the mistake of doing our own thing in isolation. As a result, we had a much greater impact on the community as a whole resulting in a dramatic decrease in the infant mortality rate.

6. **Need for economic development**. We have also learned that one often- neglected area crucial to development is economics. Through the years we have attempted unsuccessfully to provide jobs in the delta. The economic situation in the region today is actually worse than it was in 1970. Unless individuals have opportunities to earn a livelihood, there will always be substandard housing, poor sanitation, inadequate educational opportunities and health problems. Together, these culminate in hopelessness, stagnation and the creation of an underclass in American society.

The challenge for us today is to involve Christian businessmen in the development of jobs for the poor. The door stands wide open in our country for an economic mission program. We need Christian businessmen with a vision to establish job opportunities for the poor as part of an economic evangelistic mission venture. These work opportunities must be part of a total person ministry involving counseling, teaching in work responsibility and money management and other people-building programs. Without this approach, we will be unable to make the progress necessary to enable people to move into self-sufficiency.

7. **Advocacy**. As Christian physicians, health care professionals and development workers, we have a God-given responsibility to be advocates for the most vulnerable people in our society. Programs such as this can both directly improve the quality of people's lives and promote policy changes leading to new opportunities for the poor.

Conclusion

We began our work at Cary Christian Health Center in 1970 at a time of heightened social tension and without any United States model for a community medical mission program. Those early days were filled with anxieties as to whether we would succeed. The health needs of the delta were monumental but we struggled to find a meaningful relationship with community people in that polarized atmosphere.

The answer involved a combination of factors. One answer was found in the support of a few key whites and the relationship with a respected black Christian who became our community liaison worker. The other was in the form of medicine itself. Medical care was a positive, noncontroversial service to people in need. Our credibility was established by treating a host of sick children and providing services for pregnant mothers. People began to listen to what we had to say. Educational classes were initiated and mothers started to learn how to take care of themselves and their children.

Shortly after arriving in the delta, a respected community leader told me, "You can't teach these people anything and they're not interested in learning." He has been proven wrong. People were interested in learning. As a result we began to see a marked improvement in the health status of children. As an example, the number of babies with severe dehydration due to gastroenteritis became almost nonexistent.

Through our work in the delta, we discovered that one person with commitment to the poor, a dogged determination to persevere and a high energy level could enlist the services of like-minded community people. Together, they could make a difference. The most rewarding and fulfilling aspect of the work was to see those community people develop into mature, skillful Christian care-givers.

Another pleasant discovery was that local, state and federal agencies were delighted to cooperate with committed Christian people working at the local level to improve health care for the poor. They wanted to get a job done but were often stymied by a lack of dedicated people. We provided the dedication and expertise. The end result was a profitable symbiotic relationship which greatly benefitted the poor.

Cary is a microcosm of the needs which exist throughout the USA. There are thousands of such communities with hundreds of thousands of hurting people. The Lazaruses of this world are at our own doorstep. The tragedy is that they are not seen by the Christian community whose major focus in on third world poor.

The challenge we face is to open the eyes of Christians to a third world type poverty which exists in our own country and the necessity we have to reach these people with the compassion of Christ. We can make a difference.

Questions for Reflection

1. What are some of the issues in the struggle for human rights and justice that directly affect primary health care?

2. How do you react to the community leader who said, "You can't teach these people anything and they're not interested in learning"? What factors might have shaped his point of view? How might one help to change his perspective?

3. When is a long-term commitment desirable and perhaps even necessary to bring about a permanent change in community health care?

4. What are some of the socio-economic changes that often cause the development of an "underclass" in certain areas?

5. What are the family issues (single parent, abuse, etc.) that will need to be addressed to improve community health?

6. How can you help form a bridge and cross the gap to the poor in your community?

7. The author of this chapter suggests "an economic evangelistic mission venture" involving Christian businessmen and women in establishing job opportunities for the poor. How could this be done at the most basic levels? Would it work in your community? Why or why not?

Author's Note: If you are interested in this type of domestic mission ministry, the Luke Society stands ready to provide physicians, registered nurses and others with an intensive two-week training program, followed by ongoing consultation as to how to develop a health outreach among the poor in your area. Write to us at: The Luke Society, 1121 Grove Street, Vicksburg, MS 39180.

8

Meeting Physical and Spiritual Need: Community Health Evangelism

Stan Rowland, M.B.A.

Community Health Evangelism (CHE), a program of Life Ministry
Africa (Campus Crusade for Christ), was established to help the church in
Africa meet the physical and spiritual needs of rural people. The program
trains local villagers in the prevention of disease, the promotion of health
and how to live the abundant Christian life. Life Ministry attempts to deal
with people as whole beings not separated into physical and spiritual
dimensions. The program's biblical basis comes from Matthew 25 where
Jesus commands his disciples to feed the hungry, clothe the naked and visit
the oppressed. Later, he tells them to go and make disciples of all people.
That is the intent of this Community Health Evangelism program.

This case study describes a CHE project in Buhugu, Uganda. The
lessons learned from this experience have shaped other Life Ministry
programs elsewhere in Africa.

Purpose and Strategy

Project Goals

The community health evangelism program at Buhugu has several
goals:

1. To produce community health evangelists who are guided by the Holy
   Spirit and capable of reproducing themselves (in terms of their spiritual
   commitments and health knowledge) in others. Initially, the training
   team will teach health workers who in turn will train other health
   workers who will teach other health workers who will teach yet others
   these physical and spiritual concepts.

After a career in business, Mr. Rowland joined the staff of Campus Crusade for Christ in East
Africa. As Coordinator of Community Health Evangelism for more than a decade, he has
helped design community development programs and train health workers throughout Africa.

2. To integrate health development into the church's program, directed by indigenous leaders and with people taking responsibility for their own health.

3. By the second generation, to have the program totally managed by Ugandans with the program continuing and expanding into adjacent areas through a local training team.

4. To encourage the villagers to perceive the program as their own and fund its operation.

5. To gain a 50 percent improvement in the health indices such as diarrheal deaths and measles cases as compared to a baseline study completed at the beginning of the program.

6. To have one part-time Community Health Evangelist (CHE) for every 350 people (or for every 40-50 families) in the project area.

The Strategy

The program's strategy is to train Community Health Evangelists who in turn will train their fellow villagers how to prevent disease, promote good health and live the abundant Christian life. The health training includes such things as water purification, sanitation, hygiene, garden plot agriculture, nutrition and maternal/child care. In the spiritual realm, people are taught how to come to a personal relationship with Christ, how to grow in their faith, and then how they can reach others for Jesus Christ and grow in their new-found faith.

The original intent was, and continues to be, to identify and train local villagers to share their faith and health knowledge with their neighbors. This generally happens through visits by CHEs to family and friends in which they share health information and spiritual truths they have learned. They also model what they have learned and serve as resource persons to the community on local projects. Their goal is to transfer everything they have learned to others on an ongoing basis. In this way, when the training team leaves an area, the process they initiated will continue.

Background

Buhugu is a sub-county in eastern Uganda on the Kenya border, 35 kilometers northwest of Mbale, Uganda, at an elevation of 6000 feet. The sub-county is eight kilometers long and four kilometers wide, broken into twelve villages with a total population of 23,000. This is a lush and prosperous agricultural area. Arabic coffee and bananas are the main source of income. The people are industrious, exemplified by the fact that ten years earlier, one village in this sub-county was chosen by the Ugandan government in a country-wide competition as the second-best parish in development.

Beginnings

Mission: Moving Mountains (M:MM), a new, U. S.-based Christian development agency, initiated this community health project in 1981. It sought to establish a model community health program integrating physical and spiritual concerns. Life Ministry became involved when it provided two nurses for the project during the period of transition between the departure of one M:MM missionary family and the arrival of their replacements. Life Ministries continued to staff the project for the next few years.

The project began with M:MM missionaries working to build relationships with these communities. Following a series of discussions, ten communities formed health committees in each village to guide the activities that would be carried out in this project. These committees, in turn, chose twelve men — not necessarily Christians — to be trained as community health workers who would be responsible to promote health in the region. The workers answered to the committees. Two representatives from each ten-person committee comprised a local executive committee. The chairperson of the executive committee took strong leadership for the project which was a critical factor in its growth. In subsequent projects that frequently lacked someone to "champion" the project, growth was much slower.

The initial village health worker training was planned to be 24 half-day sessions meeting twice each week. The training was about one-third over when Life Ministry assumed responsibility for the project from M:MM. Each half-day session addressed one health topic and one spiritual topic. In addition to the formal group lessons, the trainees visited homes in the community in order to build relationships and gain a better understanding of local problems and concerns.

Building a New Clinic

The community expressed a strong desire for a clinic. Life Ministry agreed to staff the clinic with two nurses if the community would provide the building and housing for the staff. The local community center, though needing major renovation, was chosen for this purpose. Half of the building became the clinic while the other half served as the nurses' residence. The people provided building materials and labor. An outside agency funded the importation of needed medical supplies and equipment. After more than a year of renovation, the clinic officially opened in March 1984.

The clinic was busy from the very beginning. The staff treated an average of 50-70 patients each day. Between fifteen and twenty babies were born each month. The program operated five child-health clinics in outlying villages to screen for high-risk babies whose parents needed nutrition training. Weekly, more than fifty expectant mothers participated in an antenatal clinic to identify high-risk cases that should deliver in the clinic or even the Mbale hospital one hour away.

In subsequent projects, Life Ministry has continued the well-baby program but not established other clinics. Clinics require a long-term commitment (10-20 years) and are very costly to operate. Currently, Life Ministry tries to initiate CHE community health programs only where existing clinics already provide curative care so Life Ministry can focus its efforts on prevention.

Operation of the Buhugu Program

Selecting An Area to Work

The project staff initially considered several areas within the Mbale Diocese of the Church of Uganda for a project site. They ultimately selected Buhugu in consultation with the Bishop of the Church of Uganda and the government's District Medical Office. They felt this location had the greatest probability of success.

Originally, Mission: Moving Mountains helped the community assess its needs and then establish community health committees to direct the project. These committees then chose community members to be trained as community health evangelists. The first group of trainees had secondary school educations. The CHEs in subsequent projects have not gone beyond elementary school.

The Training Staff

The initial expatriate training team was trained in medicine. In subsequent programs we used people having any combination of nursing, public health, agriculture, sanitation, nutrition, social work or teaching skills. We found it was far better to have people with different vocational backgrounds since varied skills are needed to make the program successful.

Community Health Evangelists

The original group of 12 CHE trainees came from ten villages within walking distance of the training location. The training sessions were held two days per week until 40 sessions had been completed. Half of each training day was spent on teaching health and development topics and the other half addressed spiritual topics. The teaching was designed to be transferable so that people who had been trained could train others who in turn would train others.

CHEs learned to teach their neighbors this new knowledge through visits in their homes. Their role is to teach in the home, assist in community health projects and have a spiritual ministry.

Our experience suggests that CHEs should serve as volunteers rather than as paid employees. The Buhugu community health committee initially decided to pay the CHEs. However, they never paid more than half of the first month's salary. They had expected the profits from the sale of medicines through the program to pay the CHEs but this did not happen because they were unable to make a profit.

The community planned to sponsor fund-raising activities to support the program. This failed. In some villages, however, the people remunerated their health workers in kind (by helping with their gardens, etc.). This is one way of rewarding CHEs for their work.

In 1985, the committees chose the second group of health workers, in this case 24 women. Few could speak English. The newly-opened clinic absorbed much of the Life Ministry staff's efforts. Although responsible for training the new CHEs, the staff had little time to accompany them on home visits. Language problems further complicated these home visits since the expatriate training staff did not speak the local dialect well.

From the start, Life Ministry intended to replace the expatriate training staff with the most effective CHEs from the project. Three CHEs who had served as translators were subsequently trained to become trainers. They have helped to train additional CHEs in their area as well as in another location. The hope is that this local training team will expand the program into adjacent areas within the county. This has not happened so far. Although CHEs are unpaid volunteers, the project needs a full-time staff of paid trainers to grow. In the future, we hope that the fees charged to the villagers will pay the trainers' salaries but this has not yet been tested.

Financial Support

From the beginning, the program intended to raise as much of the project's support as possible from the local people. This happened at Buhugu. The community served meals for the trainees and gave the classroom for the CHE training sessions. The people also provided the labor, timber and sand for the clinic renovation and the construction of protected springs. But where local resources were insufficient for capital improvements and other expenses, outside agencies interested in promoting primary health care provided additional funds.

These monies helped to establish a revolving fund for the purchase of seeds, medicines and bee-keeping equipment. The fund was replenished when the people purchased these materials through the program. Outside monies were also used to purchase cement, roofing and equipment for the clinic. In addition, UNICEF provided cement, water pipes and technical assistance for protecting springs.

Results

These two training sessions had very different results. In the first group, all twelve village health workers became Christians during their training in comparison to only six from the second group. The first group actively reached out to their fellow villagers while in the second group only the six believers were active health workers.

The first group brought over 1000 people to Christ through their personal witness and started 32 Bible study groups involving 285 people. Twenty people from these original groups started additional Bible studies involving another 100 people. The six women from the second group faithfully witnessed during clinic days to those waiting and did some limited home visiting.

The results of the efforts by the first group of CHEs were phenomenal. The community protected 40 springs and built a 13 kilometer gravity-fed water system serving 10,000 people. The clinic's statistics showed that measles in the area declined by 50 percent and diarrheal deaths by 30 percent. Over 60 families began keeping bees as a source of income. A number of the CHEs started their own fish, tree and poultry demonstration projects. All improved their own gardens and built improved pit latrines.

The first group of CHEs, from all accounts, was successful in helping to meet the physical and spiritual needs of people in the community. What they learned was also transferred to other local people whom they had trained. The second group was far less successful.

We attribute this difference in success to the high percentage of the CHEs in the first group who became Christians. They also wanted to grow in their faith. In other Life Ministry projects where fewer village health workers accepted Christ, fewer people continued in the program. In two other communities, a higher percentage came to a personal relationship with Christ and more remained faithful to their tasks.

A second factor contributing to this difference in results, we believe, is the time that the trainers spent with the CHEs. The Life Ministries training staff spent more time discipling the CHEs in the first group and accompanied them on more home visits modeling expected behavior. In other projects committee members accompany non-English speaking CHEs on home visits in order to interpret for the training staff. We see these non-English speaking CHEs doing home visiting successfully with lives being changed physically and spiritually.

Lessons Learned: Integrating Physical & Spiritual Ministries

We have found it much easier to integrate physical and spiritual ministries in theory than in practice. Through this project, Life Ministries has learned several lessons:

1. **Changed lives**. Our goal is to see transformed lives as a result of inward changes through the transforming love of Jesus Christ. This inward change should then lead to physical change in individuals, then family, and then community. This has happened in the Buhugu project.

An example will illustrate. One of the first contacts we made in one community during a home visit was with Samuel, a 92-year-old man. We shared the plan of salvation with him through the *Picture Book Four Laws*. He accepted Christ as Savior. Afterward he danced around with the *Four Laws* in his hand shouting "my visa to heaven!" He then told us that he was usually drunk by this time of day (11:00 AM), but for some unknown reason on that particular day he did not drink. He now understood why. Later he became a very active committee member, helping to establish the village health program in his community.

2. **Christian trainers**. We found that the training team should consist of mature, born-again Christians. The CHE volunteers are not required to be Christians but the training begins with what it means to be a believer. If, however, the training team members are not mature Christians, it is difficult to model what is expected for the CHE.

In one project, several CHEs were not believers so could not share Christ in a personal way. People in the community asked why they should become Christians when the CHEs did not.

3. **Integration of physical and spiritual concerns**. If a community health program wants to address people's physical and spiritual needs, members of the training team must understand both. They must be able to teach basic health principles as well as spiritual concepts. This includes knowing how to win individuals to Christ.

In one of our first projects in another area, the members of the training team with the best understanding of health and development issues taught these topics. The most effective teachers of spiritual matters addressed those. As a result, two of the trainers concentrated on health issues to the exclusion of any teaching of spiritual concerns. This example suggested to the CHEs that it was unnecessary to integrate physical and spiritual issues in their teaching because those training them did not.

Both physical and spiritual concerns were addressed equally in Life Ministry's teaching. There is a danger that CHEs spend all their time meeting highly visible physical needs at the expense of the spiritual. In one community, we focused our teaching on agriculture because of the presence of two agricultural specialists on the staff. They emphasized agriculture during two, two-week training sessions with local farmers. The farmers participating in the seminar were taught how to share what they had learned with other farmers. We discovered that they shared agriculture information but none of what they had learned in the spiritual realm. Neighbors taught by these farmers applied this agriculture knowledge but we saw no spiritual change or growth.

4. **People teach the way they are taught**. A major goal of this project was for people to transfer what they themselves have learned, to other people. CHEs, we learned, will teach the way they are taught. When the

trainer stood up and lectured, the CHEs would lecture during their home visits. When we posed problems and led group discussions, so did the CHEs. If the trainer did not make home visits, neither did the CHEs. If CHEs did not dig pit latrines or make gardens, neither would the people. To help the CHEs teach more effectively, we ultimately prepared a number of picture booklets on health development and spiritual topics so they could teach more easily.

5. **Aids to learning**. In the Buhugu project, we used a picture booklet called the "Four Spiritual Laws" that described how one can become a Christian. Experience showed that the use of this booklet helped CHEs bring people to Christ. However, they found remembering what to teach about diarrhea much more difficult.

Initially, our training methodology emphasized lectures, songs, demonstrations and dramas. Later, we switched to a problem-posing focus. Learners were given the opportunity to discuss the specific problems in their community. This greatly stimulated discussion and encouraged people to better remember what was taught. This orientation toward the discussion of problems, combined with the picture books, greatly improved the CHEs' teaching. In other projects, we emphasized problem-posing teaching but this alone was not enough. However, when we combined the problem approach with picture booklets for health development topics and spiritual truths, we had much greater success.

6. **Building momentum**. Large-scale outreach programs such as the "Jesus Film" and "I Found it!" campaigns create excitement and enthusiasm for evangelism. This is also true for building momentum for development through community projects. This gives the CHEs an opportunity to make contacts and quickly build many new relationships.

In one community, church members participated with CHEs in a training program on how to share one's faith and follow-up on new believers. This was followed by a house-to-house visitation campaign in which the trainees shared the good news of Jesus Christ. At night the "Jesus" film was shown. More than 400 people became Christians during this ten-day campaign. Many joined the church. This generated great excitement for evangelism and showed everyone that Jesus Christ was a key element in this program.

A similar program in Buhugu combined evangelism with a clean water campaign. The CHEs helped the people of one village protect a spring. From there, it spread to a second village. Interest for clean water through protecting springs grew. During an 18-month period, ten villages protected over 40 springs without assistance from the project's training staff.

7. **Expect and inspect for change**. Unless we expect spiritual change to occur, all we will see are some physical changes which we believe are not usually long-lasting. If we expect spiritual changes, we should be inspecting to see that they happen. This contributes to the growth of excitement and momentum. Having the CHEs set goals and then report the results can help. The program's momentum increased dramatically after we instituted a reporting system. The same was true in areas where the trainers accompanied the CHEs on home visits in order to track physical and spiritual changes as a result of the project.

As these concepts have been applied, we have seen transformed lives. People, families and communities are more healthy, both physically and spiritually. It is our desire to see this happening throughout Africa.

8. **Home Bible studies**. Home Bible studies have been an important outcome of this program. Initially, these are led by the CHEs but then new believers start their own Bible studies as they learn and grow. The content of the Bible studies needs to be based on aggressive evangelism and discipleship principles that encourage the members to apply what they learn.

In Buhugu, all twelve original CHEs became Christians through the program. They started 32 Bible study groups using audio-tape training materials and "Picture Book Four Laws" provided by Life Ministry. These participants in turn started over twenty more Bible study groups combined with aggressive evangelism. Ultimately, over 1000 people became believers as a result.

The Future of Community Health Evangelism

Life Ministry's goal is to establish several community health evangelism projects in conjunction with the local church in each of 20 African countries. These are designed to model how the church can integrate a community health program with evangelism and discipleship. The plan calls for each Life Ministry project team to work in an area for 3-5 years, establishing three different projects. During this time, they hopefully will have helped train 150-200 CHEs in a 25-village area serving 30,000 to 50,000 people. The goal is also to leave behind a training team made up of local people to extend the concept throughout the region.

The major expansion of this strategy began in 1985 after an evaluation of the pilot projects in Uganda and Kenya. The strategy appears to be sound. The courses for training the training teams, committees and CHEs have been developed and tested. To this point, Life Ministry has twelve training teams in East Africa. These teams have helped establish seventeen projects that have trained more than 375 community health evangelists. We have planned other projects and pray that our experience will motivate other groups to institute community health evangelism programs.

Community Health Evangelism is a strategy whose time has come. People are excited about the physical and spiritual changes that result. Lives are being changed in the communities where we have training teams. Many churches and local agencies want to learn how they can establish their own integrated community health and evangelism programs. This can happen all over Africa and then on other continents.

References

Rowland, Stanley, and Don Meyers. "Are the Participants Christian?" *Together*, No. 12, July-September, 1986, pp. 31-34.

Rowland, Stanley. "Training Local Villagers to Provide Health Care." *Evangelical Missions Quarterly*, Vol. 21, No. 1, 1985, pp. 44-50.

Rowland, Stanley. "Multiplying Health and Light." *Together*, No. 6, January-March, 1985, pp. 9-12.

Questions for Reflection

1. Why do you think the CHE program picked up momentum after the CHEs began to set goals and report their results? Does accountability usually help us practice better stewardship? Why or why not?

2. How do you feel about the fact that some of the original people chosen to be trained as community health workers in this project were not Christian? What might be the dangers of this? The advantages?

3. One of the goals of this project was integrating "health development into the Church's program, directed by indigenous leaders and with people taking responsibility for their own health." What kinds of standards might be used for evaluating such a goal?

4. The goal of the CHEs to transfer everything they have learned to others on an ongoing basis might be supported by what scripture?

5. Why do you think this program found it better for the training staff to include people with varied vocational backgrounds, rather than all medical professionals?

9

Hospitals and Community Health: An Issue of Complementarity

Pakisa Tshimika, M.P.H.

The landrover lurched into the village after a dusty, bumpy three-hour drive from the Kajiji Hospital. As we climbed out of the vehicle, villagers dashed out to meet us. After the exchange of customary greetings, the village health worker told us they had a problem here — many of the villagers had been suffering from diarrhea for several weeks now.

A problem indeed — but whose problem? Who would do something about it? The hospital? The community health team? These questions are the focus of this case study of a health development program in rural Zaire.

Defining the Problem

In the past, "community health" has often been reduced to health maintenance activities, performed by professionals in the community rather than the hospital. Our community health staff at Kajiji, Zaire is seeking to rethink the concept of "community health" to mean a healthy community: a community that knows how to achieve and maintain physical, environmental, spiritual, mental, social and economic health. As we reevaluate our concept of community health, we must also look again at our community health activities. It has been some time since we were content to go to a village every month or so to weigh and vaccinate children as our contribution to that community's "health." Our question now has become, where does community health stop?

The hospital, on the other hand, has been functioning traditionally as a center for treatment of the sick. It has also served as the second step (after

Trained in public health, Mr. Tshimika served for a number of years as the Health Coordinator for the Mennonite Brethren hospital, nursing school and community health program in Kajiji, Zaire. A leader in the community health development field in his own country, he is currently completing his doctoral studies in international health in the U.S.

the community dispensary) for most people seeking health care. While treatment of the sick is a necessary function, this situation has a two-fold problem:

1. The vast majority of personnel and budget is directed to the curative services. As a result, even in the hospital context, health promotion and disease prevention — aspects of health care — have to some extent been neglected or forgotten.

2. A great deal of expertise and financial resources are invested in treating minor illnesses which normally do not require this level of care.

Do the hospital and the community health program need each other? In Kajiji, we experienced excellent results from our vaccination campaigns against communicable childhood diseases. Elsewhere in Zaire, preventive health programs have dramatically reduced intestinal parasites. Rural health posts now provide essential services to a large percentage of the country's population. However, children still become ill with meningitis; adults still suffer strangulated hernias. Community health has not prevented all illness.

We need a good working relationship with the hospital so that we can refer these cases. We need the hospital for its technical support as well as for the feedback it can provide to the community health program. We also need to build on the trust and good reputation enjoyed by the mission hospital in the community.

The question has another side: does the hospital need community health? How can community health programs assist the hospital? If we are truly interested in serving people, we must admit that the hospital leaves a wide range of problems uncovered. In many developing countries, people come to the hospital again and again for the same problem.

The hospital's outpatient dispensary provides a common example. A dispensary chart shows that a child has been treated repeatedly for hookworm. Through a local outreach program, the hospital could help communities see the causes of their health problems. They could also learn how to prevent them.

In the case of the village with the outbreak of diarrhea, the community health team helped the villagers pinpoint the problem. Every time it rained, the water washed across the animal enclosure and then down the hillside where it contaminated the primary water source for the village. Once this was understood, the village corrected the situation. The hospital provided oral rehydration solution and advanced treatment for more severe cases of dehydration when necessary. Without a community health outreach, the hospital would have simply continued to treat case after case of diarrhea.

Hospitals and community health programs need each other. Hospitals can:

● Serve as referral centers for outlying health centers and health posts.

● Provide technical services that local health centers cannot offer.

● Give community health workers valuable information about local problems based on cases referred to the hospital.

Community health services can also serve the hospital in important ways:

● Prevent disease in the community. This reduces the hospital's work load and allows it to concentrate on more serious problems.

● Provide follow-up care in the community after patients are released from the hospital. Hospitals cannot provide that service.

● Help the staff see how the hospital is viewed by the community. This makes it easier for the hospital to improve its services.

Another dimension of the problem is that of training health care personnel, both professional and auxiliary. The matter of training raises several questions in relation to mission hospitals:

● Who should be responsible for training? Is this the task of the hospital or of the community health program?

● Are the health care personnel to be prepared to work in the hospital or in the community? Where should the emphasis be?

● Where does the church fit into this program? Does the hospital exist to help the church? Is community health there to support and generate income for the church? Or is it the other way around? Do health care programs and the church need each other?

● If health programs and the church need each other, what should that relationship look like?

Some of these questions will be debated for years to come. Rather than attempting to provide conclusive answers to these questions, this case study will document the experience of the Kajiji health program. It will suggest some lessons that we learned in the process.

We realized from the beginning that community health could not survive without the hospital. Similarly, the hospital, for its part, could not provide holistic care without community health services. Hospital and community health programs are not two mutually exclusive entities, operating independently of each other. Neither should they be competitors. By integrating hospital and community health services, they can become complementary, harmoniously serving the community.

Understanding Integration

Dictionary definitions of integration speak of "coordinating" or "blending" things into functioning or unified wholes. The goal of the Kajiji health program, we decided, was to provide health care for the whole person. Therefore it seemed only logical to approach this in ways that promote unity instead of bringing division. In searching for integration, we found it helpful to think of it as a process rather than a goal.

This demands a commitment to a process, rather than an orientation toward completing a set of tasks. The time orientation is thus long-term and ongoing rather than short-term. Integration is not a one-time, limited-scope project; it must continually build on itself as it brings more and more aspects of the community's life under its umbrella. At the same time integration will not simply happen because we desire it. The work of setting objectives, planning interventions and evaluating progress is still necessary. The integration process is like a Chokwe proverb: "...a little chick, you run after it too fast, you miss it; you run too slow, you'll never catch it...."

Steps Toward Integration

Kajiji, a mission station in southern Zaire, provides medical services to around 84,000 people in Bandundu Province through three institutions:

- Hospital
- School for training auxiliary nurses
- Community health program

The Zairian Mennonite Brethren Church owns and operates these programs although limited subsidies are received from the government. The hospital work started in the early 1950s, the nursing school in the mid-1950s and the public health program in the mid-1970s. From the beginning, however, hospital personnel undertook some public health related activities.

The original decision that led us to integrate the hospital and the community health program came in response to a problem. The division into separate institutions created an attitude of "we are the hospital," "you are public health," "they are the nursing school." At times these institutions seemed to be operating autonomously, duplicating some services while leaving gaps in other areas. At times they competed for loyalty, funds and clients.

These attitudes of competitiveness and exclusivity crept up on us without our knowledge. Other people brought these to our attention. We also began to see the problem reflected in our nurses' training program. We knew that something had to be done. Many of the nurses graduating from our program were unsure what to do in the rural health posts. Some tried to create miniature hospitals, not understanding their roles in health prevention. After examining the situation, we realized that we needed to change several things:

- More harmonious relationships between the different arms of our health care program.
- Smoother functioning departments.
- Better services for the community.
- Improved stewardship of limited resources.

We decided that a carefully developed health policy would help make this happen. We set out to create one.

Adopting a Health Policy

The hospital, community health program and nurses training school followed routine. The programs ran the way they did because that was how things had always been done. When changes were proposed, it was usually because someone thought of a better way. Only seldom were changes consciously related to a guiding policy. Therefore, one of our first tasks was to formulate a policy statement for the church's medical work. The policy statement of a church-sponsored health care program, we felt, should reflect both its commitment to the Kingdom of God under the Lordship of Christ as well as its relationship to the purpose and mission of the church. The initial part of our policy statement (translated from French) states:

"Being a Christian medical work, we are not only concerned to promote the health of individuals as defined by the World Health Organization, but we also put the accent on the spiritual need of the person in following the example and the commandment of Jesus Christ as indicated in the Gospels. In our Christian compassion we seek justice in the distribution of care to the people. We believe that the medical work is also a means of evangelism and spiritual nurture for the personnel and the client."

The policy statement continues by spelling out the program's purpose and general goal in terms of promoting a state of health for the individual, the family and the community in the regions of the Mennonite Brethren Church in Zaire. Specifically it endeavors to do so through:

- Community health activities in the region.
- Providing primary and curative care services.
- Training personnel at all levels.
- Integrating health care with spiritual care, community development and nutritional work.

Setting Objectives

This health policy became the basis for setting objectives for the hospital, the community health program and the nurses training school. Each institution accepted the health policy statement and agreed to a common strategy. The next question was, how should we do it?

First, we examined the function and purpose of each institution and looked at how each could develop its potential according to its purpose. We then set objectives for each program and established guidelines for how each unit would relate to the others. Next, we identified ways through which each could support and complement the other without dominating or using each other. And finally, we outlined the strategy through which we planned to attain our objectives.

Evaluating the Existing Organizational Structure

One of our first objectives required a look at the way the hospital, community health program and nurses training school had been operating and interrelating. We realized that our attempts at integration would be difficult if not impossible without reorganization. We looked for several things in developing a new structure:

- Mutual accountability
- Support between the institutions
- Flexibility for future program development

This evaluation process led to the formation of a coordinating body to give leadership and direction to the Kajiji health program.

The Coordinating Body

We planned for a coordinating body that would represent all of the institutions involved in the Kajiji health program. This coordinating group was commissioned to facilitate the exchange of ideas, suggest improvements, and evaluate activities. In this way, each institution shared its plans, needs and concerns. Together, the staff also discussed ways through which the different departments could assist each other in meeting the common goal of improved health in the community.

Experience showed that we needed one person to coordinate this process. Someone had to balance the best interests of each institution, and not simply promote one's own activities. Someone had to facilitate communication between each aspect of the health program and with the church. In addition, the situation required a liaison with the various government representatives who followed the program with great interest.

The first step in organizing this group was to prepare job descriptions for the coordinator and members of the coordinating group. We scheduled weekly planning and coordinating meetings with staff from the hospital, the community health program and the nurses school. We discovered that when these meetings became irregular, problems and misunderstandings soon emerged because of inadequate communication.

Building a Support System

An essential aspect of working toward integration is the support system. Without an extended and committed support system, these efforts are bound to fail. We found that several groups of people must be involved in supporting integration. If they are not part of the process, they will most likely block efforts.

1. **Church leaders.** In many parts of the developing world, church leaders lack a clear understanding of primary health care. The concept of integration, we found, was generally a new concept to them. However, our church leaders proved to be enthusiastic once they understood the purpose and goals of the program.

2. **Government agencies.** Those involved in church-based health services often prefer to carry on without consultation with government agencies. This happens where antagonism between the state and the church has been a problem. This is also true where government agencies have not met their responsibilities to those implementing health care programs. Christian health professionals, however, have a responsibility to carefully study the government's policies, strategies and plans if they want to impact the health of the nation.

Although the potential for conflict is often high, government agencies are potential partners in the quest for health. We struggled to collaborate with government efforts wherever possible without compromising either our professional commitments or our commitments to the Kingdom of God.

3. **Funding agencies.** Funding agencies must clearly understand the mission and objectives of the program. Sometimes funding agencies send subtle messages with their money: "if you want our money, you must do it our way." Having clear policies, goals and objectives, has enabled us to maintain supportive relationships with our donor agencies. Those disagreeing with our mission purpose and ministry goals know they have no place in our program.

4. **Personnel.** As a church-based program, we are often approached by different agencies who wish to send us personnel. Both sending agencies and their people must be sympathetic to the policies and objectives in order to serve effectively. In particular, they must accept the principles of integration. Without this understanding and commitment, even highly skilled persons may bring division and competitiveness into the program. Thus, we found it imperative to be sure that the sending agencies are committed to support the integration process.

5. **Nurses in training**. Changes at the organizational level must also impact the training of future health care workers. Several years ago we reworked our nursing school curriculum to expose our graduates to a broader concept of health. Instead of focusing only on the traditional areas of patient care, laboratory skills and work in the maternity, we expanded our training. Our students now implement community surveys, evaluate programs, plant gardens for nutritional rehabilitation programs and have become involved in community health programs in the village. They are enthusiastic about this opportunity.

6. **The health care staff**. In our experience, it has been essential to spend time with the hospital staff and those working in rural health posts and centers. Many feel threatened by this new, broader perspective of health. The "new" nurses sometimes intimidate the older staff. We have worked hard to help the latter feel valued for their knowledge and many years of faithful service. They also need to participate in the integration process. Otherwise, they may become alienated and sabotage the process. An aggressive continuing education program for nurses, we found, helped to resolve this problem.

7. **The local community**. People in the community never hear the words, "Integrated Health Care Services." Nevertheless, they recognize that the health care delivery system at Kajiji is changing. They like it. Without their support, we would undoubtedly fail.

Imposed ideas are rarely accepted. We see the community as a partner in the health care system. People provide us with valuable feedback when we are prepared to listen. We cannot work independently of them or expect them to passively receive our ideas. At Kajiji, the integration process was clearly assisted by local leaders who never understood the divisions we as health professionals made between curative and preventive programs. They did not distinguish between the roles of the hospital, the community health program and the nurses training school. As Atkins says in this volume, health professionals need to adopt the holistic view of health already held by indigenous people.

The Basis for Integration

Our experience suggests that a successfully integrated health program requires several things:

1. **Relationships**. As important as program goals and objectives might be, they should never take priority over people. Building personal relationships is an integral part of the process at each step. This takes time — often much more than our North American colleagues are willing to commit.

2. **Teamwork**. The integration process becomes more difficult when individuals are more interested in promoting their own programs and

perspectives than collaborating together as a team. We try to give all team members opportunities to share their own ideas and experiences. This has raised morale and encouraged everyone to share in the common task.

3. **Well-equipped leaders.** Successful integration requires strong and well-equipped leaders in each part of the program. Weak leadership in one area reduces the effectiveness of that part of the team. It may then become a tool of the other areas rather than an equal partner. Each leader must be committed to the integration process as well as to the aspect of the program for which he is responsible, if the organization is to carry out its mandates within the health policy.

4. **Coordination.** Whenever this coordinating group was weakened for any reason, we found that the integration process was also weakened. The various aspects of health care began to drift apart once again becoming independent. Misunderstandings, lack of communication, wasted efforts, and failure to serve our community appropriately were the results. Weekly meetings, even without an agenda, helped us keep the integration process in focus and to solve small problems as they arose.

Roadblocks and Pitfalls

We do not claim to have the best formula for integrating a hospital and a community health program. The process is not particularly complicated. It can, however, be difficult if one does not anticipate some potential roadblocks. These roadblocks, our experience suggests, are more relational than organizational.

The qualities that make for successful health professionals also contribute to the problem. Most people involved in health development are highly committed and motivated people. They want to see God's work done *now*. They desire to save lives, prevent disease and see people made whole. They also value a job well done. These qualities become liabilities when strong commitments and high motivation lead to struggles for power.

Our task is to empower other people, encouraging them to take initiative and responsibility for their own development. Our own commitments and motivations must find their outlet in ways that do not control or manipulate people but rather help them find their place in the cooperative effort. Those of us in health development are also people of vision. Our visions, however, can become struggles to build "personal kingdoms." Although we relate best to our own visions, we must also be willing to share the vision of those with whom we work. Sometimes we focus on our differences — ideas, opinions, methods, etc. — to the extent that they become barriers to a successfully integrated health program. The shared task of helping people develop their gifts and take responsibility for their own development is much more important.

The Scope of Integration in Kajiji

We are still in the process of integrating community health and the hospital program in Kajiji. We have encountered setbacks but have also made advances. The community health program integrates a variety of activities. These include maternal-child health clinics, supervising rural health posts and centers, training village health workers, organizing continuing education for rural health post nurses, nutrition rehabilitation and education, agricultural and gardening projects, small livestock projects, training of extension agents, and road work. The community health program works with the hospital in nutrition rehabilitation and education of specific cases as well as a developing program of tuberculosis control.

The hospital personnel assist in the training of village health workers and provide continuing education for rural nurses. They provide technical supervision for the rural health centers. We hope to further involve hospital personnel in the program, making more use of their technical skills in the community as well as in the hospital. The nursing school is intensely involved in all aspects of the community health program as well as hospital work. Likewise, the personnel of the hospital and the community health program are deeply involved in the training of student nurses.

When a community has a problem now, whose problem is it? It is our problem — all of us. And we all share in its solution.

Questions for Reflection

1. How do you answer the question: "Where does community health care stop?"

2. How can hospitals assist community health programs? How can community health programs assist the hospital? Where should the emphasis be and why?

3. Do you think churches should be involved in health care programs? Why (or why not)? How?

4. Why are ideas rarely accepted when imposed on a community from outside?

5. What are some of the dangers of a lack of coordination in an integrated health care program?

6. What different kinds of activities could possibly become part of the services of an integrated community health care program?

10

Control, Influence and Community Health in Bangladesh

W. Meredith Long, M.A.

"I visited the home of a village man and his wife who had just delivered a healthy baby boy. They had wanted a boy for a long time.

"I said to the man, 'Now you must feed your wife rice, fish and vegetables, not just rice and salt.' He said, 'Yes, I'll do that.' I said, 'Bring it now and feed her before I go.' They brought the food and with every mouthful, it seemed as if the woman was choking. She had at last pleased her husband and given him a son. Now she felt she was killing the boy. She was sure his cord would not dry out and he would swell up and die. I had never seen anyone under such mental pressure. I almost told them to go back to their rice and salt.

"Later, I saw the man and asked, 'Did you continue to feed your wife everything?' He said, 'Yes, what else could I do? The things that you fed her at first would have harmed her so much that I decided that the damage was already done. That is why I kept on feeding her.' In the end, both her health and that of the baby were excellent, much better than was usually the case." (Muriel Scott, community health nurse in Bangladesh)

Health and Human Relationships

Lasting changes in health-related behaviors emerge from the dynamics of human relationships. To know who in the community controls or influences whom, is vital. Social structures illuminate the exercise of control and influence in many relationships. In other instances, the relationships may be far more subtle. In the previous anecdote, Muriel Scott drew

Formerly Asia Director for MAP International, Mr. Long worked for a number of years in Bangladesh as a trainer and health consultant. He is currently doing his doctoral research in international health while serving as health education specialist for MAP International in East Africa.

on her status as an expatriate nurse and the relationship of trust she had developed with that family to help them overcome the very strong fears associated with the adoption of this good health practice.

This chapter will examine the impact of control and influence over decisions to adopt new health behaviors in a community health program in Bangladesh.

Community Health in Bangladesh

The LAMB (Lutheran Aid to Medicine, Bangladesh) Hospital is located in a rural area of northwestern Bangladesh, a few miles from the small city of Parbatipur. The project primarily serves small farmers and agricultural laborers organized into *paras*. *Paras* consist of 20-140 homes clustered together. Several *paras* make up a village which may spread out over several square miles. The *para* rather than the village is the functional unit for the project.

Because LAMB Hospital was not required to offer community health services to all in the area, project leaders decided that only those *paras* making a significant corporate commitment could join the program. The original plan called for health committees in each *para* to oversee the project. The committees were to select community health workers to be trained in preventive health care and take responsibility for promoting health in the area. The idea of establishing a cadre of community health workers was soon abandoned. Instead, project leaders trained members of the health committees and made them responsible for an aspect of community health. One, for example, would oversee community sanitation and water supply. Another would provide prenatal and postnatal family education and so forth.

Through this process, the health committees retained a significant role. Everyone agreed from the start that these committee members would serve as volunteers rather than paid staff. Agency workers often develop good relationships with villagers at the beginning of a health project only to see them later disintegrate into arguments over payment of community health workers. By depending upon volunteers, LAMB Hospital sacrificed their ability to hold the village workers strictly accountable for specific tasks and responsibilities but also removed a major source of contention. It proved to be a good trade.

Because the project offered hospital and clinic support, the health committee members neither carried medicines nor provided curative care beyond that possible with local resources. The program focused on disease prevention and health promotion through health education in the community.

The program accepted "village doctors" and traditional birth attendants (TBAs) as allies, not competitors. Village doctors practice an elementary form of "western" medicine dependent upon medicines available in local shops. Homeopathic practitioners and Hindu and Muslim religious healers who practiced health based upon systems and values incompatible with those of LAMB Hospital were not invited to participate.

Program Methodology

The project team began working in *paras* by sharing health information on community problems. During the course of several visits, they presented health lessons using highly participatory teaching methodologies. Following these sessions, community members met to determine whether or not to participate further. If they decided to continue, they were required to select a health committee to receive more in-depth training.

Early in the program, the village health committee members studied a fixed curriculum. The project's training staff soon abandoned this in favor of a more flexible approach.

The new curriculum consisted of eight, self-contained units highlighting the eight health practices through which individuals and communities could most improve their own health. The program emphasized practical actions. Each health committee member had to demonstrate proficiency in some practical skill (i.e. mixing oral rehydration solution) before moving on to the next unit. The order of the lessons varied from person to person and *para* to *para*, reflecting different needs and interests. Committee members learned to teach others in the *para* and apply their simple skills when problems emerged in the community.

The project's goal during the first year was for each person in the *para* to hear and understand eight basic health lessons. In monthly meetings, the project staff encouraged the health committees, advised them on their health education work and provided additional training. Every three or four months, several health committees met at the hospital for further training, sharing experiences and special activities such as health dramas and films.

At the end of the first year, the *para* had to demonstrate community support for the program by requesting that it continue. In most cases, communities saw significant progress in the eight health areas during the first year. As the program expanded into other development activities, community motivation and interest increased.

Integrated Components

Other health activities not directly linked to the work of the committees nonetheless reinforced and shaped the LAMB program. As a result, the program also improved people's health in *paras* where no health committees existed or where they were ineffective. Having a variety of activities raised staff morale as well. Something was always "going right" to provide encouragement when other things went wrong.

The community health program included several elements.

1. **Curative services**. The hospital provided outpatient clinics from the inception of the project. In-patient services followed within a couple of years as the hospital was completed and staffed. The hospital also initiated a mobile clinic program. The mobile clinics did not come to the *paras* that had health committees but did visit areas accessible to those *paras*. Health committee members therefore did not find their credibility undermined by the frequent appearance of medical professionals. Access to curative services was still inconvenient enough to motivate preventive and promotive behaviors.

2. **Nutritional programs**. The hospital established a feeding program for malnourished children, supported by project teams conducting growth monitoring of children in the surrounding communities. In *paras* with health committees, committee members coordinated the nutrition program and weighed and monitored the children's growth through "Road to Health" charts.

3. **Health education**. Clinic workers stressed health education, even in the curative aspects of the program. Patients in the clinic received individualized instruction in areas related to their illnesses. All clinic personnel, both clinicians and support staff, completed the same training program as the health committee members. Therefore they knew what was being taught in the communities and could provide support to the health committee members responsible for implementing the program.

Program staff also provided health education in the local schools. Children were less resistant to change and so could reinforce what was being taught in the community. The project's community health staff with the assistance of committee members conducted special health exhibitions in local bazaars and in the communities. These special events — dramas, films, demonstrations or health games — generated widespread participation and considerable excitement.

Some program staff, for instance, took a series of slides in the villages and sequenced them to tell a health story. Reflective question and answer sessions flowed easily into lively, group interaction following the slide shows. Program staff members were also renowned for their dramatic skills and developed plays which presented good health behaviors. Again, reflective questions followed the dramatic presentations.

Project personnel also monitored the health education messages broadcast over government radio. While LAMB Hospital had no direct ties with the media, exposure given to such subjects as oral rehydration over the radio reinforced the project's teaching.

4. **Village doctor education**. At the start of the project, no one anticipated the close cooperation between the health program and the village doctors. The staff wanted to neutralize possible opposition from village

doctors in the immediate area so invited them to participate in the training program. Surprisingly, most of the doctors not only attended the first session but enthusiastically welcomed the opportunity for further training. Since their informal medical training had not touched on prevention and promotion, they found this emphasis very interesting.

Project staff expanded their training for village doctors in disease prevention and health promotion. Many doctors subsequently began to emphasize prevention and simple home treatment in their practices. Medically focused training also improved the doctors' medical skills and helped them recognize their own limits. They more readily referred difficult cases to the clinic or hospital.

Village doctors began functioning as auxiliaries to the hospital's health program on an independent and self-sustaining basis. Their relationship with the hospital enhanced their own credibility within the community but also increased the influence of the project staff among them. The village doctors also had a financial incentive to maintain this association since the practice of good medicine generated higher incomes than did the practice of poor medicine.

5. **Traditional birth attendant training**. If village doctors were surprisingly receptive to additional training, traditional birth attendants (TBAs) were disappointingly resistant. Whereas the village doctors valued scientific knowledge, the TBAs depended upon traditional practices and their own experience. Convinced they had little to learn from the young and less experienced project staff, TBAs saw no reason to change their birthing practices. Continuing efforts to provide the TBAs with further training largely failed. As a result, the project introduced changes in child-bearing practices in other ways.

6. **Clean water and sanitation programs**. The project also offered latrine and tube well programs. Although all *paras* were eligible for assistance, project staff specifically targeted *paras* with health committees. Members trained, motivated and organized their own villages.

The project paid half the cost of building cement latrines and most of the cost of the tube well. To be eligible for a tube well — the most attractive component of the program — 20 percent of the homes in the *para* had to have latrines. People also had to use them. The *para's* contribution to the tube well had to be raised through small contributions rather than be provided by one individual who could later lay claim to the well.

Relationships of Control and Influence

The interplay of control and influence in Bangladesh society shaped LAMB's program and continues to influence its direction. The result is reflected in several different contexts:

Family

"One woman trained in this program cooked the evening meal for her husband and went into labor. About nine o'clock, she delivered the child but not the placenta. She said to the village midwife, 'Don't do anything.' The midwife didn't listen. In the end, she put in her hand and pulled out the placenta. Within minutes, the room filled with blood and the mother died. The next day we went to the *para* to teach. During the class, a little child walked in and asked, 'Where is my Mommy?' It was the child of the woman who died the night before."

"Another woman was brought in. Her baby had already died but the mother could not deliver, so she said to the midwife, 'Don't do anything. Let me go to the hospital.' The midwives said, 'No, that is okay. We can do it.' Three or four midwives together tried to pull out the baby. Some pushed from the outside, some pulled from inside. In the end, they gave up and sent her to the hospital." (Muriel Scott)

Teaching only expectant mothers about childbirth was not fully effective. They often exercised no real control in decisions regarding their own deliveries. The husbands, however, while culturally barred from actually attending the delivery nevertheless played a critical role as decision-makers.

"People believe that pregnancy and childbirth are women's concerns. But we found so much darkness in the area because men have had nothing to do with it. Education makes such a difference. Men are the ones who tend to be educated. They read, see and hear things so the key for us now is working through the men."

"We ask the men, 'Do you know what is happening? Aren't you responsible for your wife? Don't you care?' The men are completely amazed; they do care what is happening to their wives and children. They say, 'I am not going to let the midwife touch my wife again.' So the midwives are pressured by the husbands into changing. That is why they are changing." (Muriel Scott)

Although the men still do not attend deliveries, their expectations of cleanliness and care have changed. Because of their authority within the home and control over the reimbursement to the midwife, they can force changes which otherwise would not happen as quickly.

The extended family as a group plays a role in decision-making going beyond the authority and influence of any one member. Significant changes in behavior are based more on group decisions than the result of individual choices. Therefore when project staff visit a family, other members are encouraged to come and hear the message.

"If we tell a mother after delivery, 'You must eat everything,' she can agree but it is a waste of time unless you also teach the husband and mother-in-law.

"It is much better if other people are present and understand. Otherwise, the minute we leave, they will say, 'Don't listen to what they tell you.' If we teach the mother outside her village, she will listen and do what we say. But when she returns home, she has to interact with a lot of other people."

"Her husband will say, 'Don't do that to the baby.' Her mother-in-law will say, 'Don't do it.' Her neighbors will say, 'Don't do it.' You have to make sure that within a given community, *everybody* understands what needs to be done." (Muriel Scott)

Village Authority

The formal process through which *paras* became part of the health program emphasized community ownership. The project initiated the first few health education sessions in a village. The process only continued, however, if the *para* decided to move ahead and issued a formal invitation to the project staff to work in their community. The *para* then elected a health committee and selected people for training.

Some communities decided not to participate — a decision the project staff respected. Communities could also withdraw from the program. After the first year, each *para* evaluated its experience with the program and decided whether to participate further. Those health committees or communities that lost interest dropped out.

Status and authority in the community also affected the selection and role of health committees. Since committee members were unpaid and uncredentialed, persons of higher ascribed status within the community were rarely appointed to the role. If selected, they were less likely to continue than were those of lower social status.

Since health committee members enjoyed few of the perquisites associated with high ascribed status, they had to "prove" their competence to community members. Consequently, the training program tried to enhance their status by emphasizing practical skills that visibly benefitted the community. When a community's first activity in the program succeeded, this success affirmed the health worker's credibility and status and encouraged the community to move ahead with new initiatives.

The decision not to attach high status to the health worker's role through formal credentials, salaries or distribution of medicines benefitted the program in another way. Committee members had little opportunity to market their services in other communities. It was easier to replace an inactive incumbent with someone new. Health workers were not "fired" in the usual sense. Those lacking the qualities of concern, service or enjoyment in teaching and learning usually dropped out on their own. Those possessing these qualities tended to succeed.

Indigenous Medical Practitioners

Earlier we noted that the significant role of indigenous medical practitioners ("village doctors") made this project unique. Village doctors practiced medicine before the project began and would undoubtedly continue doing so after it ended. Many sincerely tried to provide good health care to their communities. Initially, project leaders merely wanted to neutralize any negative influence village doctors might exert over the project in the community. Soon, the staff recognized these indigenous healers as an important part of the health care team. This partnership with the village doctors worked for several reasons:

1. **Respect**. The community respected village doctors for their role in delivering health care services. The project staff reinforced this feeling by affirming their contribution to people's health.

2. **Training**. The LAMB Hospital staff presented village doctors with opportunities for further health training as a "professional courtesy." No one approached the training of these indigenous practitioners as if they were failures or deficient. They themselves determined how they could benefit from this training.

3. **Avoidance of competition**. The project-trained community workers were unpaid, did not distribute medicines and did not compete with traditional village doctors. No permanent clinics were established. The mobile clinics began only after the project built a strong relationship with the village doctors. As a result, the latter were not threatened by the mobile clinics.

4. **Increased credibility**. The project staff accepted referrals from village doctors and provided good care. This enhanced the doctors' credibility and improved the quality of their service to the community. It also increased their willingness to refer difficult cases to LAMB Hospital. Referrals were therefore less likely to be perceived as deficiencies or failures by either the village doctors or their patients. This responsive referral system strengthened the relationship of village doctors to the project.

Power of Outside Agencies

Outside agencies often provide resources and services otherwise unavailable to a community. The staff of external aid organizations, particularly health care professionals, usually command high respect and status in Third World communities because of their credentials and access to resources. This combination of status and resources usually gives expatriate workers significant power in the community. The use of that power, even unintentionally, significantly affected the project.

Striking a Deal

"Everyone was very keen on getting tube wells but not so keen on latrines. So we said that 20% of the homes in the para had to have latrines before a community was eligible for a tube well. We gave them the tube well at a very reduced price...but we insisted that everyone contribute a small amount. That way, no single individual could claim it." (Muriel Scott)

Although relatively successful in this case, the approach in which an outside agency dictates terms to the community by controlling access to the program's inputs raises several questions. Does the agency know enough to set reasonable conditions? Is this "enforced development" (latrines in this case) linked with education? Is there follow-up (such as training in the maintenance of latrines)? In its use of power, does the agency become an ally of the powerless or a friend of the powerful? Does the program maintain a balance between community and agency initiative, resources and responsibility?

Providing Services Without Establishing Mastery

"One thing we learned was the importance of providing clinic facilities. When someone is seriously ill, they really do need curative care. On the other hand, we didn't want to make medicines too available. When we started the mobile clinic program, we did not locate it directly in a community health *para* but rather nearby so the people could benefit from its services without being tied to the program." (Muriel Scott)

In addition to the clinics, the LAMB hospital also operated feeding programs for those with special needs. These were structured, however, so as not to compete with community responsibility. The program struggled to balance two concerns; providing needed outside resources and yet allowing communities to develop and carry out their own initiatives. The issue becomes particularly sensitive when it involves restricting access to services desired by the community. The physical distance of the LAMB hospital from the community helped to preserve community involvement.

Do it! It's Good for You!

"Paternalism" is a dirty word in development circles. However, fear of appearing paternalistic may prevent an occasional and careful use of authority, within a relationship of mutual respect and trust, to bring about needed change.

"The village doctor said they must bathe the patient to keep the fever down and must give him food and drink. The family was horrified but agreed and said, 'But you must stay with us the whole time we bathe this child and give him something to eat. If anything goes wrong, then you will be here.'" (Muriel Scott)

As in the incident which opened this chapter, the key to overcoming the high, perceived risk of adopting new behavior was the person and authority of the health care professional. Experience in this project suggests that several things are necessary for the successful exercise of authority within a helping relationship. This requires a sincere desire for the other person's good, a regard for the dignity and worth of the other, an attitude of humility and a relationship of trust. In a paternalistic relationship, good intentions are not enough to overcome a lack of dignity, humility and respect.

Sharing Status

Health professionals often undermine the credibility of indigenous health care providers. Through their attitudes and actions, professionally trained health workers often communicate the message that the practitioners of traditional medicine are incompetent and not to be trusted. LAMB hospital reflected a different attitude.

"One day I received a note from a village doctor asking me to come and see him. He had a patient with diarrhea. I nearly did not go. I thought that since he had treated people with diarrhea longer than I had, he probably knew better ways of treating them than I do. But something made me go. When I arrived, he did not want me to treat the patient. He had already told the patient to keep on eating and drinking. The relatives were so horrified that he asked me to come and support what he said. I was really glad I had gone just to support him and say 'yes.'" (Muriel Scott)

Health professionals with credentials must use their status to support their competent but less well-trained colleagues.

The Authority of Love and Respect

"Don't be scornful of what they believe. That is true to them. They have believed it a long time. Do not make them feel stupid because of what they believe. Say, 'Yes, I know you believe this. Why do you? Let's think about it.' They, themselves, must think, 'Yes, we should change.'

"I really love the villagers. They are lovely, lovely people. If you care for them, you really want them to change. Even though it's slow, there is really no need to get impatient with them." (Muriel Scott)

Extraordinary programs are the result of extraordinary people. Love and respect rooted in a high valuation of people is a necessary foundation for building helping relationships. Spontaneous and natural declarations of the loveliness of villagers made without condescension are, in my experience, however, rare enough to be remarkable. I suspect that manipulators of relationships of control and influence are distinguished by the community from respected, interpersonally skilled partners in change less by their specific actions than by what motivates and underlies their actions. The

LONG   97

capacity of a follower of Christ to break down resistance to change by force
of steadfast love and patience should be a major distinctive of Christian
health care programs.

   The LAMB project staff modeled wisdom, respect and love in their
relationships to the villagers and village doctors involved in the health
program. In so doing, they encourage and challenge those who would
presume to help others in the name of Christ.

Questions for Reflection

1. What attitudes are helpful for the successful exercise of authority by a
   health care professional when encouraging the adoption of new health
   behaviors in a community?

2. Why is it important that health care professionals do not undermine the
   credibility of indigenous health care providers?

3. What are the strengths and limitations of working with indigenous health
   care practitioners in promoting health development?

4. How do you feel about the issue of payment for community health
   workers versus depending on volunteers? What might be some of the
   advantages and disadvantages of each?

5. What kinds of attitudes inside families might need to be changed in
   improving community health care?

6. The project in this chapter found it helpful to use highly participatory
   teaching methodologies. Describe some of the characteristics of a participatory teaching style.

11

Community Health: From Delivery to Responsibility

Richard Crespo, Ph.D.

Few people had latrines. None bothered to wash their hands before eating. Many children continued sick as before.

The six-year project was half over and little had changed. The community health project staff realized that something had to change soon. They carefully evaluated their services and training programs. Everything appeared to work as planned. The project served more people than ever, services were provided on time and promoters were well-supervised. Everything was working well, so why were people not changing?

The staff concluded that they must not be doing enough community education. They beefed up the education program. They poured money into film projectors, portable generators and films. The staff reorganized their work in a way that freed up more time for teaching.

The films were a smash hit! People flocked to the education programs. Success waited just around the corner. Yet, as time passed, behavior remained unchanged. Hardly anyone built latrines. No one washed their hands before eating and the children remained as sick as before.

How can community health workers facilitate behavioral change? Lack of response to educational initiatives frustrates many development workers. Some project leaders cope with this frustration by searching for new educational strategies and methods. Others increase the size of their program's educational component. Many criticize the people for being unwilling to improve their lives.

Dr. Crespo worked with Intervarsity Christian Fellowship in Central America before initiating MAP International's Latin America program in Ecuador and becoming MAP's first Regional Director. He is now director of MAP International's Health Training Resources department in Brunswick, Georgia.

Educational methods are inadequate solutions to this problem. As the example just cited suggests, education often has little impact on people's behavior. The reason many health education programs fail may be caused by the way project staff view the health education process. Health professionals bring a service delivery orientation. Yet, the evidence suggests that community-based health care is more appropriately based on a facilitation of development orientation.

The shift from a service delivery orientation to one of facilitating development involves a major learning process. This chapter presents the case of a project in South America struggling to shift its orientation from the delivery of services to the facilitation of community health development.

Project Background

In the mid-70s, Quechua Indians in the South American Andes requested medical services from a nearby Christian mission. The mission had little experience in rural health care so they asked MAP International to help design and implement a primary health care program.

Since 1975 the project has touched over 100 communities and trained 142 local leaders in disease prevention and health promotion. Today, nearly all of the communities in the project are part of the Ministry of Health's (MOH) primary health care system. At the request of the MOH, project staff continue to help provide supervision and continuing education to the government's community health workers (CHWs).

Service Delivery Orientation

The project began with minimal outside resources. The training staff donated their time. Community health workers paid their own way to the training sites. Equipment was held to a minimum. Communities desiring to participate in the program were required to raise the equivalent of U.S. $50 for a small stock of medicines and equipment. They built a room for treating patients and committed themselves to implement environmental improvement projects.

A year after the project began, external funding became available. The staff began relying on outside resources to the exclusion of what could be raised locally. The external funds enabled the project to expand its coverage but the requirements for local responsibility were loosened. Because of the project leaders' genuine concern to help as many people as possible, communities were allowed to participate in the project without meeting the basic requirements.

The project staff assumed that community members could be motivated to become responsible for their health by simply offering health services. They defined their project outcomes in terms of the numbers of people that used health services. The project had a service delivery orientation. The project staff did not involve local people in analyzing community problems but they told the CHWs what needed to be done. They also trained the local health workers to do it. The project staff focused their attention on program administration.

The CHWs learned to promote immunizations, build latrines, protect water sources, clean houses, organize communities, etc. However, their mode of operation consisted of providing these services in response to requests from the people. People were expected to do as they were told — and sometimes they did — while the CHWs delivered health care services to the community.

The project staff intended to develop people but their service delivery orientation resulted in emphasizing infrastructure and services. They defined outcomes in terms of numbers of health services. The more complete the range of services offered, the better the program was assumed to be.

Three years of experience led the project staff to become dissatisfied at two levels:

● The project's services depended upon resources from outside the communities. The staff foresaw the day when additional outside funding would no longer be available.

● People were not responding to the educational programs. The CHWs diligently taught their weekly health classes. The staff purchased projects and portable generators in order to show health films in the communities. People flocked to see the films but few applied the principles they were taught. Very few boiled their water, used latrines or practiced personal hygiene.

Development Facilitation Orientation

Dissatisfaction with the project's progress stimulated the staff to rethink their strategy. At first, they searched for new and more effective educational methods and techniques. The breakthrough came, however, when the staff discovered the difference between the *service delivery model* of community health and the *development facilitation model*.

A project following the delivery model concentrates on the effective delivery of services. The development facilitation model, in contrast, emphasizes the fact that people must learn to take responsibility for their own well-being. The project staff realized that effective primary health care emerges when people learn to act in ways that promote good health.

This shift in perspective changed how the project staff regarded the role of CHWs in the community. It also led to a new view of the health education process.

Development Initiators

CHWs changed the way they did their jobs. Instead of delivering services, they became community initiators. They learned how to challenge people to reflect on their lives and how to help them analyze alternative solutions to local problems. The CHWs stopped waiting for people to come to them. They initiated interaction with people, challenged existing patterns and encouraged people to change.

For example, the brother of Manuel, a CHW, built a barrel to catch rain water from the roof of his house. His neighbors commented on this unusual device but continued to draw their own water from the contaminated pools at the bottom of the gulch near the center of the community.

During a family visit, Manuel noticed the rain barrel and immediately grasped its potential. He observed something that was already going on (but outside the program) and began to discuss it with the community. He challenged people to think about their own contaminated water supply. Manuel also set an example by building one himself. Soon a few neighbors followed suit. Slowly over the course of a year, rain barrels appeared throughout the community. The people regarded it as their own idea!

The community now responded to Manuel because he changed his approach. Instead of spending most of his time at the health post, he put a priority on home visits. Early in the morning before people left for work, Manuel would visit as many homes as possible. He realized that home visits were the culturally acceptable way to build relationships and discuss important personal matters.

Additionally, the project staff no longer decided which community projects would be implemented. They encouraged Manuel and the other CHWs to initiate projects as people expressed interest and concern. This process complicated the project administration because not everyone was working on the same project at the same time. On the other hand, as in Manuel's community, people acted out of genuine interest, not simply because resources were available.

Listeners

The project staff and the CHWs also changed the way that they taught health. Instead of simply transferring information, they learned to listen. No longer did they consider health education merely as giving a health talk or showing a film. They learned to listen to the community's concerns and to design educational experiences where the people make their own decision about what to do.

Specifically, the CHWs implemented a strategy with four components:

• Sharing health information
• Reflecting on this health information

- Planning health actions
- Practicing health actions

The CHWs began by stimulating the residents' imaginations with information regarding local health problems. Having captured interest, they then opened discussions about these problems. Sometimes these discussions lasted a few minutes, other times they continued for months. As the people articulated these problems, the CHWs began directing the discussion toward plans for solving them. Finally, the health workers facilitated action by encouragement, by example and by drawing on available resources.

The key to the educational strategy was the CHWs' ability to ask questions and listen. It required nearly a year of intensive training for the CHWs to master these basic skills. At first, the CHWs asked a few leading questions and then gave up. Unable to tolerate silence, they stopped asking questions and began lecturing again. The breakthrough came for the CHWs when they learned to ask the people about their experiences. The CHWs would then reiterate the problems mentioned by the people and ask for possible solutions. The community would then come up with their own solutions instead of waiting for answers from the expert.

Alfonzo, one of the CHWs, told of "preaching" for months in his own community about the importance of latrines. Individuals would acknowledge the truth of what he said but never did anything about it. He became so discouraged that he wanted to quit. Just in time, the project staff began training Alfonzo in the skills of teaching through listening and asking questions.

Later as Alfonzo learned to listen, something happened. Suddenly it seemed as if everyone wanted a latrine. He became so deluged with requests for advice and "professional approval" that he was again ready to quit. He felt that he was being overworked!

Alfonzo discovered a secret. The radical change in attitudes came when he began, for the first time, to listen to his friends and neighbors' concerns. He discovered that people rejected latrines because they were afraid that their little children would accidentally fall through the hole in the floor! Once Alfonzo became aware of the problem, he was able to help the community residents think through ways to solve it.

Once everyone expressed their feelings openly, Alfonzo could help them confront their fears. Interestingly enough, Alfonzo's previous training had desensitized him to the perspectives of his own neighbors. In order to be effective and get back in touch with his own people, he had to change his stance from that of a health professional, to a stance of an encourager and listener.

Conclusion

The project staff found it difficult to shift their orientation from service delivery to the facilitation of development. As health professionals, they had a strong temptation to do things that were actually the responsibility of local people. They found it frustrating to wait until people were ready to take action. The difficulty in making the shift was due to the fact that a shift in orientation requires fundamental changes in how health programs are structured. Service delivery and the facilitation of development differ from each other in terms of their purposes, processes and personnel.

Purpose

In a service delivery orientation, the purpose is to deliver services. Initially, the project staff defined their project outcomes in terms of numbers of health services. They believed that people's health would improve as a result of the existence of services. With this kind of purpose, the staff did not think to wait for community members to take initiative. Delivery goals had to be met.

In a development facilitation orientation, the purpose became to mobilize people. While health services were necessary, project outcomes were assessed in terms of the initiatives that local people took to improve their health. A tension existed in that project staff could not predict or control how people would mobilize. For example, project staff had funds designated for latrines while community members were busy making rain barrels.

In this case, the purpose of the project became that people take action on activities of their own choice. Health services exist to support and encourage community initiative.

Process

Service delivery and development orientation differ in the process used for promoting change. In the beginning project, staff concentrated their time on management and administration. They thought that their goals could be accomplished through efficient management of resources and personnel.

In a development facilitation orientation, the project staff realized that the fundamental process is dialogue. Facilitating development became a matter of spending time with people in reflection and analysis. In the end, people changed when they acted out of personal and collective commitment. And project staff discovered that a key to starting dialogue was to ask people to talk about their experience.

Personnel

A third way in which service delivery and development facilitation orientation differs is in personnel. In the former, project staff relied on CHWs to conduct project activities. Community members were expected to go to the CHWs and were the ones who implemented project activities.

Later when the orientation shifted to facilitating development, project staff realized that the key personnel were the community members. Anyone could learn the essential skills, and everyone should be responsible for community projects.

When health projects rely only on delivering health services, the danger exists that people will become dependent on others doing things for them. The challenge for all community health workers is facilitating people into taking responsibility for their own health.

Questions for Reflection

1. What are the different emphases of a development facilitation model in contrast to a service delivery model of community health?

2. What are some of the motivations that make it difficult for health care workers to wait until the local community assumes responsibility for its own health care?

3. What are some of the dangers when health projects rely only on delivering health services?

4. What is it that effective facilitators do to promote behavioral change?

12

Saradidi: Community-Based Health Development in Kenya

Dan C.O. Kaseje, M.B., M.P.H., Ph.D.

Today, not a single malnourished child from the locations covered by the Saradidi Community-Based Health Program can be found at the Lwak Nutrition Rehabilitation Center in the Siaya District, Kenya. For nearly a century, the Lwak Center has struggled to improve the health of the people of Siaya with few tangible results. This community had one of the highest rates of infant and childhood mortality among all the districts of Kenya. More than 20 percent of the children died before their second birthday. Children inundated the health center. Most children improved on admission but many relapsed as soon as they were discharged.

The main causes of death in the community included measles, diarrhoeal diseases, acute respiratory infections and malaria — all preventable diseases. The Saradidi community health program changed all that. Infant mortality dropped from 181 per 1000 live births to 89 per 1000 live births in just a few years. Other indicators suggest that health in the community has improved significantly.

What brought about this success in the Saradidi program? Not mobile clinics. Not more experienced doctors or specialists from North America or Europe. This milestone was achieved by the cooperation and participation of the community at the grassroots level. Though poor and uneducated, these people helped to wipe out malnutrition and significantly reduce child mortality. These goals were accomplished long before more sophisticated medical technologies such as anti-malaria prophylaxis and community-based treatment of malaria were introduced in Saradidi.

Formerly a Lecturer in Community Health in the University of Nairobi Medical School, Dr. Kaseje then served as Project Manager for Kisumu Primary Health Care Programme of the Aga Khan Health Services in Kenya. An internationally known consultant in community health development, the author is currently Director of the Christian Medical Commission in Geneva.

Saradidi Rural Health Project is a community-based program emphasizing the prevention of disease and the promotion of health in Western Kenya. Organized by the Development Education Program of the Anglican Church (Church of the Province of Kenya), the project has mobilized the community to improve the health of people through education and development. This chapter will describe how the Saradidi Anglican congregation defined local problems, established priorities and organized and implemented the program.

Background

The project is located in Nyanza Province's Siaya District near Lake Victoria in Western Kenya. More than 90 percent of the people in the District are subsistence cultivators. Ethnically, Nyanza Province is inhabited mainly by the Luos, the second largest ethnic group in Kenya. Around half of the population is under 15 years of age. Rapid population growth has exerted much pressure on the land, depleted the soil and caused erosion. The adult literacy rate stands at about 50 percent. The population in this area numbers approximately 50,000.

The health status in Siaya District is generally poor. At the onset of the project, the infant mortality rate was 181 per 1000 live births. More than half of the community deaths occur in children under the age of five. Malaria is the most common frequently-treated health problem in the area. Measles, diarrhea, vomiting and malnutrition are responsible for high morbidity and mortality rates. Health services are inadequate and often inaccessible to people in the community. The situation is further complicated by poor transport services.

Goal of the Project

The Saradidi Anglican congregation decided to initiate a program that would mobilize the people to promote health and development in their own community, and particularly to reduce and control malaria. The program included three major goals:

1. To mobilize the community to identify its own resources for the program and sustain the program over time.

2. To encourage the people to learn about health, change their attitudes toward health (particularly malaria) and adopt new health behaviors.

3. To reduce the morbidity and mortality of people in the community.

In addition, the project was set up to develop training materials for community health programs and to assist the university in training social science graduate students to develop and implement community health programs.

It was felt that this program would be more effective if it involved the community in all health activities including specific medical interventions like oral rehydration therapy and immunization of children. Effectiveness would be measured in terms of utilization of the services and reduction in morbidity and mortality.

With some help from outside facilitators, the people of Saradidi organized themselves to participate in solving their problems. They discussed their health problems, developed a consensus on priority needs, identified available resources, explored possible solutions, implemented disease control activities and evaluated the results. Community participation was both a "means" and an "end." This was considered the best means for solving health problems, but in addition, was viewed as critical for developing a self-reliant community.

Project Planning and Implementation

The project was organized by villages in order to reflect existing structures such as geography, religion, kinship and administrative boundaries. Age and social status were important factors for well-accepted leadership roles in Saradidi. The local leaders chosen for the project were mostly over 45 years of age and the wealthier members of the community.

Conditions favorable to community participation included the fact that program ideas were initiated from within the community and decisions were taken at traditional community meetings open to all residents. The community was also reasonably homogeneous and able to mobilize and use local resources. Outside resources were available for training, for family planning services and for malaria control. However, the contribution of the community was never overshadowed by the external resources. Community needs were readily identifiable and there seemed to be an openness to change. Religious affiliation was also a strong bond in the community and helped provide a commitment to voluntary work for the good of others.

Although the initial idea of the project came from the community, the detailed planning was done with the assistance of health professionals who also grew up in the community. The group planned activities necessary to implementing the project. These included:

● Problem identification (community diagnosis).

● A community workshop to verify the results of the community diagnosis and set priorities.

● Assembling resources (staff, money and materials).

● Implementation of specific actions decided on by the community.

● A system for monitoring and evaluating the project.

The program was built on several activities — mobilizing the community, training Village Health Helpers (VHHs) and providing chloroquine for malaria prophylaxis. It was believed that this would reduce mortality and morbidity and motivate the community to take additional actions. This, in turn, would motivate VHHs to spend more time and effort in providing training and other health supplies to the community. The community, meanwhile, would provide local resources to support the efforts of VHHs.

The Saradidi Project included both the scientific methods for disease control activities and the social-cultural patterns of community participation. Since the community was effectively involved at every stage, the project activities and methods were suitable to local needs and conditions.

This development project as planned by the people was not a research program. However, a research component was built into the program to complement community efforts and to document lessons learned for other projects in the country and region. The Department of Community Health at the University of Nairobi provided the technical personnel for the research. The Kenya Medical Research Institute also helped provide equipment, supplies, transport and staff for research activities.

The baseline data, gathered in August, 1979, collected information concerning:

- Environmental conditions
- Availability of health service
- Immunizations in the community
- Nutrition status and food availability
- People's knowledge and attitudes regarding health and information about local health practices
- The practice of family planning in the community
- The demographic and economic situation of the area

This survey formed the basis from which progress was to be measured. It also helped to identify areas where health interventions were needed.

Training

Community participation in health care often involves volunteer community workers. First, a group of "trainers" was selected and trained in Saradidi. They, in turn, trained the Village Health Helpers (VHHs). By 1984, 126 VHHs had gone through some training. The community was allowed to select its own VHHs without predetermined criteria. Of those selected, 97 percent were women, 99 percent married and 75 percent between 25 and 40 years of age.

The community decided that the program would accomplish more if the VHH would train local people after they completed their own training. Leaders and other community members could participate in the training if they wished, though the training was not designed for them. The training had four aims:

1. To help VHHs identify and respond to the important health problems present in their villages, avoiding abstract concepts and generalizations.

2. To teach *specific skills* needed for *specific situations*. For example, "How do I prepare oral rehydration fluid for a child suffering from diarrhea?"

3. To respond to and build upon community needs and perspectives. The trainer began with problems that the VHHs and the community had identified and could do something about, such as sanitation. The trainees agreed to go and do a particular action at the end of each session.

4. To develop the empirical analytical skills appropriate to each village by teaching analysis of common village health problems, the appropriate information needed in the situation, the reason the problems occurred, and what could be done. Theoretical concepts and intellectual strategies were avoided and a "common sense" approach adopted.

Participatory training was considered high priority by the community. The process of training was continuous and suited to local problems, perceptions and resources. Training methods and materials were made deliberately flexible to fit the age, education and social status of the trainees. Training was done in or near the villages where the participants belonged. Later evaluation indicated significant changes in the trainees' knowledge, practices and behavior. The VHHs spent 5 - 10 days each month on the project and were more effective when they were responsible for less than 50 households each. VHHs trained by fellow VHHs performed as well as those who had been taught by trained trainers. The Saradidi training model now forms a major part of the national guidelines for the training of community health workers in Kenya.

Outcomes

The results of the project can be seen in the following discussion of objectives:

Objective 1: To document the process of community organization and involvement and measure its impact on utilization of services.

The community was organized into three areas based on the degree of involvement in project activities. These areas were further divided by villages based on geography, clan and administrative boundaries. VHHs in two areas were supplied with chloroquine starting in May 1982. The third served as the control group.

Each village selected a Village Health and Development Committee (VHDC). By the end of the first year, many of these were "dead" or weak. Their roles were taken over by the Central Committees and project staff who continued motivating and supporting the VHHs.

VHHs were provided with chloroquine phosphate in both tablets and syrup to give to all symptomatic persons who came requesting treatment. In the first area, the VHHs also provided chloroquine phosphate to pregnant women for chemoprophylaxis. This system was backed up with education regarding prevention and treatment of malaria. The community's knowledge and practice changed remarkably between the first and second surveys.

In the first survey in April 1982, most people were obtaining antimalarials from local shops. After May 1982 most people went to VHHs in their villages for chloroquine. The drugs supplied by the VHHs were always available and accessible to the community and the VHHs well informed regarding dosages. The drugs were also affordable. Hence one can conclude that the VHH system made chloroquine available, accessible, affordable and acceptable to the community and people were more willing to complete the course of treatment.

The project has now developed a self-financing scheme which enables the VHHs to supply drugs and other commodities indefinitely. The user of the system now meets the cost of services provided. Although the VHHs are not now the most popular source of drugs, they are second only to clinics. The system continues to function well. During the past eight years, only four of 126 VHHs have dropped out; two moved away, one was removed by her village, and another stopped for personal reasons.

Objective 2: To measure the impact of the community-based project on mortality.

Between 1981 and 1985, mortality rates by age, sex and area were measured by household registration of vital events. These were recorded by household visits by a team every six to eight months.

Morbidity rates were difficult to define. Problems were encountered with the VHHs measuring of birth weights: measurement was done at varying intervals after birth, not all newborns were weighed and when weighed, the forms were often filled out incorrectly and weights recorded inaccurately.

The Saradidi experience showed that an integrated comprehensive approach is the most effective in reducing mortality and morbidity. Major killers such as measles, diarrhea, acute respiratory infections, malaria and malnutrition are all interrelated. Intervening against only one will not have much effect.

Objective 3: To assess the impact of the community based program on the knowledge, attitudes and practices of the people about malaria.

Four surveys (1979, 1983, 1985, 1987) were carried out to determine the outcome of this objective. Knowledge about causes of malaria increased over the seven years from 30 percent to 50 percent. The practice of some preventive methods increased from 58 percent to 92 percent. No improvement in the proportion of houses with mosquito protection was noted. This may have been due to economic reasons.

Objective 4: To assess from time to time, availability of resources within the community to enable the program to continue indefinitely and to document which community factors were vital for the program's success.

This assessment was done through surveys and periodic project reviews at community meetings. The VHH was confirmed as the major resource. The best ones even became trainers of new ones.

Voluntary group participation was another resource sustaining the program to a large extent. Most of such participation came from women and church groups who initiated many of the health promotive activities. Harder to measure but still very real was a feeling of ownership. This roused in the community a desire to see the program succeed.

Surveys done in 1986 indicated several problems. The VHDCs which were supposed to form the village leadership were often weak or non-functional. This involved lack of communication with the Project Central Committees and project full-time staff. The VHDCs also faced management difficulties perhaps due to a lack of training. This was later realized to be a big omission in the project implementation strategy.

Technical problems also came up particularly in relation to village-based activities such as choosing a site for the construction of village wells and the selection of income generating activities. In their enthusiasm, communities sometimes selected ambitious, ill-fitting projects which could not be managed with the available skills and resources. Failures discouraged the people. External factors such as drought leading to famine in 1984-85 affected members, who had to spend more time and energy struggling to survive and less time in community activities.

A community workshop in August, 1986, helped community members review their performance and set new objectives and strategies. This self assessment was an effective community-motivated tool. The workshop showed that the community can monitor and evaluate its own work but needs encouragement to carry on.

Evaluation

The main objective of the five-day workshop for the community in 1986 was to review the situation, compare it to what had been planned in 1980, and then strategize for the future. Participants were divided into three groups with directions to list the benefits of the project as well as its past and present problems.

Benefits

The assessment found that the Saradidi health project brought a number of benefits to the community:

- Accessible health services and maternity care at the village level
- New knowledge regarding health, nutrition and disease prevention
- Immunizations for preventable diseases
- Introduction of new agricultural practices
- Training in health development and skills of tailoring, carpentry, poultry production and water protection
- Improvement in the general health of the community

Problems With The Project

During the early days of the project, the community experienced a number of problems: withdrawal of a health insurance scheme (that had been part of the project), lack of adequate communication between villages and the project staff, lack of locally available agricultural supplies (drugs, tools, etc.), lack of adequate clean water and inadequate transportation for the project staff.

Looking to the present, the community mentioned things such as the high price of chloroquine, the lack of financial support for the village health helpers and the ineffectiveness of some local development committees. Some people also noted the lack of adequate water supplies, poorly maintained roads and inadequate health services at the local level.

In general, participants recognized more benefits than disadvantages from the project activities, and their problem list was shorter than expected.

Each group of participants was then asked to assess the implementation of the program using the following questions:

1) What have we done as individuals or groups towards the achievement of program objectives?
2) What observable changes have taken place?
3) What did we set out to change that has remained unchanged?
4) Why have these expected changes not occurred?

Some of their findings are listed below.

Observable Changes

Participants in these discussions identified the following improvements as a result of this project:

- Services such as immunization, first aid, antenatal care, and family planning and nutrition education are now available locally.

- People now know how to remain healthy.
- More people are practicing soil conservation and planting trees.
- The agricultural workers assist local farmers with the treatment of their cattle, poultry, and crops.
- More people have established kitchen gardens.
- More mothers participate in antenatal clinics.
- More children have been immunized.
- More people are practicing family planning.
- More homes now have dish racks, rubbish pits and latrines and make use of these facilities.
- Malaria treatment is now available in the villages.
- A flour mill and canteen have been established in the community.

What Was Not Achieved

In spite of these achievements, other goals had not yet been realized. Some families still lacked access to a clean water supply, the use of family planning is still low, and some village development committees are still ineffective. Most villages have not yet developed income generation activities or begun using artificial insemination services as a means of improving cattle production.

Why These Changes Were Not Achieved

Not all of the anticipated changes were realized, the community decided, because they involved new ideas (artificial insemination, family planning) and people change slowly. In specialized areas such as developing clear water sources, some people lacked the necessary information, skills or money needed to adopt new techniques. In other cases, some community health committees were ineffective and volunteer workers inadequately supervised. Some volunteers were described as lazy or discouraged by their lack of pay.

Next Steps

After these training sessions, participants in the workshop went out into their village groups for community analysis in making resolutions for the next five years and creating plans of action.

The community analysis indicated that members feel they have benefitted from easy accessibility of health services at the village level through the VHHs. The presence of the VHHs had led to improvements in home and environmental cleanliness as well as knowledge in preventive and promotive health behaviors. The community also indicated they had improved in their knowledge of nutrition, immunization coverage had increased, and more home deliveries were being handled by trained persons. Training was seen as the major benefit. Help was also realized from the agricultural input and technical training.

The communities indicated a lack of effective communication between villages and the project center. Their assessment agreed with others who felt that the VHDCs, which were to form the communication link, had not worked out well.

The Project Development Committee had only 13 officials and the project, a staff of eight. It was impossible for them to visit the villages often due to other heavy responsibilities and a lack of transport.

Insufficient financial support for the VHHs came up often in the discussions. It became clear that such support would not be available from the villages soon enough and so the project center tried to help the VHHs earn money through income generating activities. Other local problems — lack of water, poor roads, and lack of transport for referrals — could only be addressed through greater collaboration with other government ministries.

In spite of these problems, the participants concluded, the project brought significant benefits to the community.

The Saradidi experience has already been a major influence on primary health care policy in Kenya. This was accomplished through:

1. A booklet entitled "The National Guidelines for the Implementation of PHC."

2. Membership on the Ministry of Health's National Training Team.

3. Two manuals produced based on the Saradidi experience for the training of trainers in PHC and for Community Health Workers. These documents are used widely throughout East Africa.

Lessons Learned

The Saradidi health project taught a number of important lessons:

1. **Working within existing structures.** Our experience suggests it may be inappropriate to reorganize the community for participation in health care and to set up a new leadership system such as the village health development committees. The reason for this is that every community has a functional organization and leadership which enables them to manage their communal tasks. Such organizational systems are recognized by and are responsible to total community membership. This system is rooted in the culture of the people.

Any new organization is not only an unnecessary duplication but is likely to confuse the community. They will invariably consider it foreign and belonging to the organizing agent and hence an added burden for which they would need compensation by the external agent. The new structure will be unfamiliar, will interfere with community cohesion and thus inhibit participation. It is therefore necessary to identify the existing system, learn how it operates, and if necessary, to strengthen it. This means working with this traditional, indigenous structure as a junior partner, enabling people in the community to achieve their own goals.

2. **Task forces.** To implement the kind of program described here, the community may need to identify people to serve as part of a task force with a specific task. This group, however, should be given well-defined tasks and specific time frames within which to function.

3. **Community participation.** Participation is enhanced when activities are not concentrated in the hands of a few members who serve as health workers or development committee members. Having more people involved in the program with small tasks is more effective than having a few people involved with greater responsibilities.

4. **Obstacles to community participation.** Natural calamities such as famine may divert the efforts of the community away from development, toward the basic struggle for survival. Activities that go beyond the technical or economic capacity of the community also tend to frustrate people and undermine their confidence. This may cause them to stop carrying out activities that they could easily undertake by themselves.

5. **External resources.** Activities requiring external resources should not be embarked upon if their benefits are not tangible or realized early. People have to understand these benefits if they are to internalize these activities. The question of sustainability should always be carefully considered. Any activity that will lead to dependency on external resources must be avoided.

Much as it is necessary that the community should control everything including resources, this control should generally be limited to the resources generated from within the community. This will enhance the accountability of the leaders to their own community. Giving them charge over external resources makes them accountable more to the external agent and may undermine mutual community trust and generate unhealthy jealousy and rivalry.

6. **Income generating activities.** Income generating activities are difficult and may not work if organized in groups without an adequate support system to ensure tangible benefits commensurate with participation inputs. Most groups would need technical assistance in selecting income generating activities, marketing and start-up resources. In areas like Saradidi where most people are preoccupied mainly with meeting basic needs which are crucial for survival, it is understandable that they would not be too eager to take investment risks necessary in any business venture. The support system should be capable of guaranteeing success.

Conclusion

Our experience at Saradidi shows that communities are not only interested in participating in their own health care but are quite capable of analyzing their situation, prioritizing their problems, and deciding on action to take to solve their health difficulties using their own resources.

Implementers of Public Health Care in Kenya have all undergone training to enable them to carry out the community principles developed in Saradidi. Allowing people to become active participants in their own health care not only empties measles wards, it becomes a fulfilling process of motivating communities to become self-reliant and resourceful in meeting community needs.

Questions for Reflection

1. Name some community conditions that are favorable to the establishment of good community participation in its own health care? What might be some obstacles to community participation?

2. What are some of the factors that may prevent a community from accomplishing favorable changes in their health care?

3. Why might it be desirable to identify the existing system of leadership in a community and work within their hierarchy as much as possible, rather than imposing health care committees upon their already-existing system?

4. This chapter makes the statement: "Having more people involved in the program with small tasks is more effective than having a few people involved with greater responsibilities." Have you found this to be true in your own ministry opportunities? Why or why not?

5. What are some of the best safeguards against engendering a dependency on outside resources in community health care?

13

The Future of Medical Mission

David Hilton, M.D.

The future of medical mission promises to be as exciting as its past, but it will, however, be vastly different from that past. Not only is the image of the pith-helmeted jungle doctor long gone, but today even the concept that health depends on doctors and hospitals is being questioned.

Over the last fifty years sweeping changes in developing countries have affected all activities, including health care. Former colonies have become independent nations. Indigenous churches have become established in former "mission fields." Medical care has become increasingly technological and expensive. Enormous population growth and urbanization have added to the burden of already crowded institutions. Vast improvements in transportation and communication have widened horizons.

Medical missions have responded to these changes with the same pioneering spirit as the generations before. With governments taking increasing responsibility for health services, churches find themselves filling the gaps of what the government is not able to do, and Christian health professionals, many indigenous, are in mission working for foreign governments or corporations. Increasingly "missionaries" are sharing medical knowledge at the invitation of local churches rather than directing medical programs.

Primary Health Care

During these years an awareness developed, first among medical missionaries, that the western medical model based on one-to-one curative medicine is not the best model to deal with the overwhelming volume of illness found in developing countries. Such a model provides expensive

After more than a decade as a missionary physician with the Brethren Church in Nigeria, Dr. Hilton worked for a number of years with the Indian Health Service with the Seminole Tribe in Florida. Currently Associate Director of the Christian Medical Commission in Geneva, Switzerland, he consults and leads training seminars on community health development around the world.

care for the relative few who are within reach of institutions, but no health care at all for most persons. Some churches have begun promoting primary health care, using scarce resources to provide simple basic health care to all instead of sophisticated technology for a few. The issue is the equitable distribution of health care resources and in this area the churches are leading the way.

Community-Based Health Care

A second issue that has emerged is the dependency, created by the curative model of medical care, on the professionals and the health care system, which deprives persons of dignity and self-reliance. A response that churches have made to this problem is to use community development principles in what is called community-based health care, which helps people take responsibility for their own health.

The method is based on the fact that eighty percent of illness and death in developing countries is preventable and that even persons without formal education are capable of learning and practicing healthy behaviors. Churches already using this model deploy community developers who facilitate discussions in communities about their health problems, thereby raising consciousness about causes of illness and generating questions about solutions. The communities then form a health committee and choose a "health promoter" from among themselves to be trained in health teaching and simple treatment. Experience with this method around the world is showing remarkable results. With appropriate information and motivation provided by a trusted member of the community, self-reliance in health care is totally transforming the health of whole communities (Contact 41). For example, malnutrition and diarrhoeal dehydration, two major causes of death in most of the world, have been virtually eliminated from whole communities by the people themselves with simple, locally available materials. Expensive hospital and even clinic care is bypassed at great savings in manpower and drugs, to say nothing of suffering, while essential primary care is made much more accessible to both rural and urban populations.

Community-based health care is also a much better vehicle for evangelism than hospitals and clinics. When people are enabled to discuss their problems these are not limited to health. The most appropriate time and place for finding solutions to moral and spiritual problems is when questions are being raised in a community by its members. The most appropriate person to facilitate the findings of those solutions is a respected member of that community such as a Christian health promotor. And so in many places where this method of health care has been implemented communities have also been transformed by the gospel.

Two-Way Mission

True to the increased understanding of mission as a two-way process, the concept of community-based health care is beginning to be exported back to the western world. Serious reflection will reveal the dependence of North Americans and Europeans on doctors, hospitals and medicines for their health. Yet the US Surgeon General reports that eighty percent of illness and death is due to what people eat, smoke and drink; they are preventable. Education has had little effect on this situation. Some USA churches are beginning to experiment with community-based health activities using modifications of the model described above (Contact 77). The effect, for many western church members, is to bring medical mission to their own communities, churches and homes. Churches have been the pioneers in health care for centuries and there is every reason to believe that they can be the vehicle for urgently needed community-based health care to be established in the industrialized world.

The Congregation as a Healing Community

This movement could well lead to a maturing concept of medical mission through a new understanding at the grassroots level of the Christian congregation as a healing community. The Christian Medical Commission has held nine conferences around the world for Christians to discuss their unique perspective of health, healing and wholeness. The New Testament church has been a model of Christian life often extolled but seldom copied in modern times. Numerous experiments in Europe and America have aroused interest. One study in twenty-four Lutheran churches in Minnesota (USA) clearly demonstrated the effectiveness of congregational activities designed to improve caring skills in reducing alcoholism and its related problems among the membership (Thorsheim and Roberts, 1984).

But again it is in the developing world, where the importance of community has not yet lost out to individualism, that the concept is widely applied. The Kimbanguist Church in Zaire is a clarion example of how the gospel can transform not only persons but communities when the biblical description of the Christian life is taken seriously. In Jamkhed, India, such a phenomenon has taken place outside the confines of an institutional church. Not only have disease and hunger been controlled but the caste system, landlordism, and the oppression of women — all contributors to ill health — have been voluntarily abandoned (Contact 10).

The Role of Health Personnel

Major changes will occur in the role of the missionary health professionals with these developments. First of all, all health professionals, indeed all Christians, are seen to be in mission for Christ. Frontiers to be crossed may be cultural or economic rather than geographic. As Third-

World churches continue to mature and take increasing responsibility for evangelism in their own countries, familiarity with the culture enhances gospel presentation and Christianity is seen less frequently as a foreign religion.

Meanwhile, for us the needs at home become more apparent. The health conditions of Americans living in inner cities, on Indian reservations, and in Appalachia must be an abomination in the sight of the Lord. Courageous Christians are desperately needed, not only to step in and fill the gaps, but to raise the issue in political and economic arenas. Christian health professionals are needed to infiltrate the decision-making levels of government and business as well as medical professional organizations to raise the issues of justice as did Amos and Hosea.

Secondly, as persons worldwide are empowered to take responsibility for their own health, health professionals will be freed from large numbers of routine treatments to give adequate time to the complicated illnesses for which they are trained. Since physicians deal primarily with disease, they will need to see themselves as peripheral and supportive to the total health care system rather than central as in the currently prevalent disease cure system.

Finally, as healing communities become more common, health professionals will move from being body mechanics toward being facilitators of healing. Doctors will have a special role in mediating Christ's healing love to the many whose brokenness is manifest in physical disease.

As the world has progressed, medical mission has changed from early "jungle dressing stations" to well equipped, modern hospitals and medical schools. The current initiation of primary health care programmes using community-based activities to facilitate widespread health improvement in both developing and industrialized countries represents the beginning of a new era with widened horizons.

The concept of the church as a healing community has been talked about and written of for over a century (Harding and Lambourne). But the concept remains largely upstaged with such medical technology as triple coronary bypass, CAT scanners and organ transplants in the 1990s. The concept of Christians in mission as a healing community was an integral part of the apostolic church, demonstrating the power and love of God. The future of global medical mission lies in congregations around the world each helping each other rediscover the healing power of that love in such a vital way that the nonbelieving world will take notice and want to become part of it.

References

Harding, G. C., and R. A. Lambourne. "Health and the Congregation." *International Review of Missions*, Geneva: Commission on World Mission and Evangelism, April 1968, pp. 193-200.

"Jamkhed Project." *Contact* 10, Geneva: Christian Medical Commission, August,1972.

"Rediscovering Traditional Community Health Resources: The Experience of Black Churches in the USA." *Contact* 77, Geneva: Christian Medical Commission, February, 1984.

"Rural Basic Health Services: The Lardin Gabas Way." *Contact* 41, Geneva: Christian Medical Commission, October, 1977.

Thorsheim and Roberts. *Substance Abuse Prevention: A Social Ecology Approach.*, Minneapolis: St. Olaf College, July, 1984.

Questions for Reflection

1. Discuss the role of physicians as "body mechanics" in contrast to the role as facilitators of healing. How are they the same or different? Is one more appropriate than the other? Why or why not?

2. Do you think churches should be concerned about and involved in the equitable distribution of health care resources? Why or why not? What might some of the problems be if they do?

3. If you had to preach a sermon proposing that your church become involved in health care, what scripture references would you use?

4. How can community-based health care provide opportunities for evangelism?

5. What might a local congregation do if it wanted to become a healing community?

NOTE: An earlier draft of this paper with the same title appeared in International Review of Mission, Vol. LXXVI, No. 301, 1987, pp. 78-81. Used with permission of the World Council of Churches in Geneva, Switzerland, publishers of the journal.

14

The Church Empowered

Jose Miguel De Angulo, M.P.H., M.D.

The first affirmation of the Bible and the Christian faith is that God created the heavens and the earth. The Creator God made all things and everything comes from him, even the will of human beings to choose or reject the communion and love that the Creator offers them. Even though all nature is a reflection of his glory, power and beauty, women and men are unique because he created them in his own image.

Another basic affirmation is that human beings chose to make themselves the center of creation, putting aside their own Creator. Since then, their way of perceiving themselves, the Creator and nature has been distorted. It was the beginning of the plundering of nature and the exploitation of fellow humans. Fortunately, God was not willing to give up on his loved ones. He committed himself to restore, not only those into whom his image and likeness were poured, but the whole creation as well. He decided to give himself as a ransom to set us free from the bondage into which we were trapped.

If human beings are the image of the Creator, and if God's desire through history is the whole salvation of the whole person, the Church must be committed to the process of restoration. The real meaning of "salvation through Jesus Christ" must be proclaimed and lived. We cannot limit or fragment the most important word that describes God's activity: "salvation" (*sozo*: to heal, to preserve, to save, to do well, to be whole, to make whole). The church must be committed to the challenge of facilitating God's plan to free people from all that restricts them from coming into a right relationship with God, their fellows and nature. Poor health is a clear example of the alienation into which people may fall — alienation from God, other people, nature and the ability to work.

Dr. De Angulo worked as a physician in Colombia until concern with the condition of the poor in Latin American society drove him to further studies in Theology and Community Health. Dr. De Angulo serves as the National Director for MAP International in Cochabamba, Bolivia.

The Concern for Justice

Several chapters in this book show how social and economic structures contribute to poor health in many places in the world. Boelens, for example, suggests that without opportunities to earn a livelihood, people will suffer substandard housing, poor sanitation, inadequate educational opportunities and health problems. If we want to really proclaim the Gospel, we must seek creative ways to deal with unjust social and economic structures. Otherwise, much of the world will lack clean water, access to appropriate education and the possibility of growing or buying adequate food. They will remain trapped in a vicious cycle of poverty, marginalization and poor health. The growing gap between the "haves" and the "have-nots" is creating a complex and miserable health situation for the majority of the world's poor.

This does not mean that Third World nations will achieve adequate health only when they arrive at a particular standard of living. The major factor contributing to good health in poor nations, Mosley shows, is the commitment to equity in the provision of basic health and other social services. What a challenge to the Church! The Church can commit itself to facilitate the development of equitable social, political and economic structures. While it may not usher in the millennium, the Church's commitment to justice will demonstrate eternal values to the world.

The Church: Empowered to Restore Wholeness

Throughout the Bible, we see how God's people have received the challenge and privilege of being a redemptive community, restoring the broken to wholeness.

God called a marginal nation to be holy, to serve the Creator by carrying out his purposes and to be priests, as God's representatives before the world (Deut. 7:6-7; Ex. 19:6; Deut. 28:9-10). In these passages, one priestly role was to provide health; not simply biological health of individuals but a holistic health that implies harmony with the Creator, with others, with social and political structures and with nature. This was the meaning of *shalom*, as suggested in Atkins' chapter. God desired *shalom* not only for the nation of Israel but for all humankind. However, this is only possible through the saving work of the Creator.

Three Old Testament words help provide a better understanding of the meaning of salvation. The word "save" implies "to heal, to restore, to keep alive." The word, *Hayah*, connotes "to give full and prosperous life," "to preserve," or "to keep alive." The second word, *Go'el* means "to purchase from slavery," "to redeem," or "to set free." Finally, *Yasha'* suggests the notion of being "free, without constraint, to develop without hindrance." We can hardly proclaim the Gospel message if we do not understand and commit ourselves to God's idea of salvation throughout history.

In the New Testament we see how God's purpose of incarnating himself among humanity was to clearly show what kind of holistic salvation he was bringing and to show us the model that we are called to follow. His compassionate and holistic restoration of people, setting them free from all that may restrict, bind or corrode the dignity and quality of life, is a clear example of the salvation he was proclaiming. The ministry of healing was a key part of that salvation. It was not limited to what we today call diseases, but displayed the broader meaning of *Yasha'* in the Old Testament.

Many passages in the Gospels show how salvation implies entering into Christ's Kingdom and beginning to produce the fruits of that Kingdom (Matt 4:23; Mark 1:14- 17; Luke 4:18-21). Jesus clearly delegated to the Church the responsibility to bring God's Kingdom to all places in the world in order to extinguish the empire of death (John 17:18; Luke 12:31-32).

If the Church does not assume this responsibility for the restoration of all things, especially the brokenness of humanity, who else will do it?

In John 20:21-23, Jesus appointed the Church to be not only the "object" of God's redemptive activity, but also the "subject"; bringing God's salvation to all of humanity. The Church has been sent by the Lord and equipped by the Holy Spirit to continue what Jesus began during his ministry on earth.

It seems that the heavens were expectantly waiting for the Church to exercise her entrusted mission. Even the heavenly host cannot intervene because this great mission has been given to the Church. People need not continue living impoverished and unhealthy lives because God has commissioned the Church to be the agent of restoration. There is no longer room for fatalism. Today is the day of salvation. What Christ started in Luke 4:18-21 is continued by the Holy Spirit through the Church. That is why the Lord said that the gates of Hades shall not overpower his Church (Matthew 16:18).

The Redemptive Community

The Kingdom of Light entrusted to the Church does not have to remain in a defensive or defeated attitude before the evil, violence and destruction that goes on in the world. It does not matter how strong the gates of oppression, disease, poverty and corrupted structures may seem. God's people have received the challenge and privilege of being a redemptive community, called to restore the brokenness of humanity and nature.

We must not limit our participation to providing only care, relief supplies, or materials while witnessing a progressive deterioration of the social, moral, economic and health situation of the majority of the Third World's population. Countries and communities have been forced to adopt modernization strategies that have increased the gap between the rich and the poor. People, particularly in rural areas, face serious problems because national development strategies tend to erode the existing village economy and its traditional subsistence relationship with nature. As a result, many migrate to the cities.

In this growing urban context, people's traditional values and culture decay in the face of new problems. Crowded into slums and left destitute, many recognize their own deprivation by contrast with the extravagant lifestyles of the wealthy. These feelings of deprivation result in alienation, low self-esteem and a sense of hopelessness.

God has chosen his Church to bring "salvation through Jesus Christ", and empowered her with the Holy Spirit. Jesus' own life is the model for this mission of healing and restoration. Throughout history God has called people to present a holistic Gospel to the world.

A Holistic Approach to Health

Developing nations are experiencing a major economic and financial crisis. In many countries, the privileged classes are insensitive to the needs of the poor while local governments care little about equality and justice. Add to this a limited view of health that focuses on disease, hospitals and trained experts, and the goal of health for all is unreachable. This gives the Church a unique challenge.

A holistic approach to health care recognizes that economic and political structures are major constraints to the health of the world's poor. What is the role of the Church in this context? Will we be content to merely treat disease or will we address the economic, political and social structures that compartmentalize health and reduce it to a simple biological matter?

It is time for the Church to become priest and prophet to the world. The Church must follow the Lord's example, becoming servants to the marginalized and alienated people among us, restoring them to wholeness. When Jesus saw the paralytic man, he healed him, commanding him to arise and walk (John 5:6-8). His solution was not temporary. He did not command his disciples to carry the man around. Instead, he restored him to wholeness.

The Church must be careful not to get so wrapped up in religious activities that, like the priest who found the man beaten by robbers on the Jericho road, it has no time to respond to human need. Busy trying to please God, the priest passed by on the other side and thus missed what God expected of him. The Church is invited to follow the example of the Samaritan who was willing to seek means to fully restore the beaten man. Only then does health take on a deeper meaning for the Church. This is the *shalom* the Father has been inviting his people to bring into their communities and nations. In this environment, people may grow in maturity in their relationships with their families, communities, nature and their Creator.

This does not result from paternalistic aid, from temporary projects, or from fragmented and superficial approaches.

Shalom is something which neither governments nor development agencies can accomplish, but the local church, with the genuine Christian commitment of its members, has been empowered to bring this about.

The Challenges of a Comprehensive Approach

The whole Church will have to deal with a more far-reaching view of health than the western one if she wants to be faithful to Scripture. Holistic health will be the core of that salvation. It will not be sufficient to work in isolated activities, even though they may look great, like putting a patch from a new garment onto an old one. "Christian" activities like feeding the hungry and healing the sick are not sufficient and may even be harmful if they are performed in isolation from the overall plan of building the Kingdom and strengthening the local church. "No one tears a patch from a new garment and sews it on an old garment. If he does, he will have torn the new garment, and the patch from the new will not match the old" (Luke 5:36 NIV).

In order to embrace the Kingdom, the Church must reflect critically and then take action on such issues as the following:

- Using a comprehensive evangelism, instead of the dualistic evangelism separating words from deeds, confronting the deep influence on our society of the Greek philosophical worldview that divided things into matter and spirit (body and soul), giving supremacy to the first element.

- Discovering the kinds of impact the Church can have on social, economic and political structures which affect health issues.

- Working to achieving "do-able" solutions to socio-economic problems, promoting food production, creating jobs, job training, etc.

- Promoting a healthy family life in midst of political, economic and social distress. One of the challenges will be to present Kingdom alternatives to singles, orphans, refugees, the rapidly-increasing numbers of single-parent families and other related family issues.

- Exploring alternatives to provide, especially for the most marginal members of society, better and more accessible education, nutrition, income generating activities and comprehensive and appropriate agricultural development.

- Getting involved in the struggle for human rights, seeking to preserve human worth and dignity, especially on behalf of those who cannot speak for themselves.

Questions for Reflection

1. In what ways do you think churches in your country have been guilty of restricting the meaning of the word "salvation?"

2. What are some of the cultural and political factors involved that help promote the stubborn persistence of unhealthy individual and community behaviors?

3. Discuss the relationship between modifying unhealthy behaviors and helping people gain a new concept of themselves, which allows them to assume responsibility for shaping the quality of their lives.

4. What is the responsibility of the Church in the struggle for justice and equality at the family, community and national levels? Where and how should you and your local congregation be involved in this struggle?

15

Trends in Medical Missions

D. Merrill Ewert

The changing face of medical missions has involved some new trends that we must consider as we look to the future. While this book does not pretend to be the definitive statement regarding changes in medical missions, it has attempted to identify several central themes that are relevant to the future.

1. **Holistic health** - In the past, we focused our attention primarily on the treatment of illness. Missions provided health care to the world's poor in many countries that had inadequate health delivery systems. This gave medical missions a distinctly western emphasis on disease. Many societies have viewed health in more holistic terms — seeing health and disease within their social, cultural and spiritual context. We are now witnessing a return to this same perspective in the West — the one that existed before the dawn of modern medicine.

2. **Prevention of disease and the promotion of health** - The new health care agenda is emphasizing the prevention of disease and the promotion of health through actions taken to eradicate the conditions responsible for health problems. Activities not previously understood to involve health are now considered part of health development. The futility of treating preventable diseases on an ongoing basis, readily apparent to most health workers, has led to the development of new programs that address the underlying causes of ill health.

3. **Participation** - In the past, health programs have been community-oriented but we now see the importance of making them community-based. The significant difference is that in the latter, people are the authors of the process. They identify their own problems, invest their own resources and make decisions regarding their own health. This requires people to commit themselves not only to the goal, but also to the process itself through which community-based programs are developed.

4. **A broader development agenda** - Health is more than a medical matter. The health of a community can only be improved by a variety of local actions that address people's physical, social, economic, psychological and spiritual problems. Ill health can be reduced only as people are adequately nourished, have access to clean water and immunizations, practice good hygiene, etc. In some cases, this requires education or health information. In others, the economic conditions of the community must be improved before we can see a change in people's health. In other contexts, the underlying problems may be psychological or spiritual. Given the interrelationship of these factors which contribute to disease, health development programs must be flexible in addressing the problems of people and communities.

5. **New skills** - Historically, health has been perceived in western society as the domain of medical professionals. However, it is becoming clear that scientific skills are not necessarily the most appropriate means to address the underlying causes of disease. The skills of diagnosis and treatment are central to the elimination of illness. However, interpersonal and communication skills are more appropriate for educating people and motivating them to change their behavior, and mobilizing communities to improve conditions in the environment that promote disease.

The people skills of development — creating a caring environment, promoting discussion of local problems, exchanging ideas, challenging assumptions, building consensus and motivating people to take action — must be learned and practiced. The process is one through which facilitators help communities develop an awareness of local problems, to examine the underlying causes, and to identify and implement appropriate solutions.

6. **Focus on training** – New skills must be consciously developed through training. We expect health care workers to obtain appropriate training before they begin to practice medicine. In the same way, the skills of community health development must also be learned — communication skills, leadership skills, relational skills, teaching skills, group process skills, etc. If community-based development is part of the new medical missions agenda, training must be a central part of the process. Kaseje's experience in Kenya shows that ordinary people can develop the needed skills and significantly improve the health of a community. All people need is the opportunity and some simple training.

7. **New relationships** - In the past, we have looked to medical professionals for solutions, assuming that their technical knowledge, skills and competence would solve most health problems. This placed physicians and other health care workers in a powerful position vis-a-vis those whose needs were being addressed. These "new priests," as Atkins calls them, have not been particularly effective in solving the underlying problems that cause ill health. A community-based health development strategy, as presented by

the authors in this book, requires a new relationship with the poor and oppressed. Although we will always need specialists to treat serious medical problems, the new health agenda requires many more "facilitators" with process skills to teach, train, encourage people to change their behaviors. They will come not with technical answers but with questions that enable people to reflect on their problems and identify solutions that they can implement for themselves.

8. **New institutions** - The development of health care institutions meant that disease problems were taken out of the community and brought to the professionals for treatment. Now, the new understanding and concern with underlying causes means that we must bring the health worker back into the community to help people address these causes at the source. This presupposes new institutions — community-based programs — or old institutions with a new agenda to make this effective. Unfortunately, this has led to conflict in some areas as people committed to health have seen curative institutions and preventative programs competing with each other. In reality, the two agendas complement each other as Tshimika's experience in Zaire has shown. The issue is one of balance and complementarity. Everyone recognizes that serious medical problems are the proper domain of curative institutions. However, hospitals and clinics must turn to preventive programs to eliminate the conditions that cause ill health.

9. **Concern for justice** - The social, economic and political conditions are ultimately responsible for, or contribute to, the prevalence of ill health and disease. Increasingly, the Church is recognizing its prophetic responsibility to speak out against injustice and challenge the government to meet the needs of its citizens. In other cases, it may be necessary for the Church to help provide basic social services that are necessary for health and wholeness.

10. **New geographical areas** - Western churches have historically viewed medical missions as something that occurred overseas. One went to Asia, Africa or Latin America to find human suffering and treat disease. We now realize, however, that even industrialized countries have underserved populations — hidden peoples — with unmet health care needs. Increasingly, leaders from the Two-Thirds World are suggesting that modern missions in the West must begin at home. "Don't come here and tell us how to solve our problems before you address your own." Boelens' case study clearly shows the tremendous need in North America and suggests how these can be met.

The basic principles of health development were first identified and refined in rural communities. With rapid urbanization around the world, more energy must be directed toward finding viable solutions to the problems of the city. If the Church really wants to promote health and wholeness among the world's poor, it must give more effort to building effective urban development models.

11. **A spirit of collaboration** - We have sometimes assumed that western missions must solve the problems of the world. Since the West controls much of the world's resources, we have also tended to define its problems, develop strategies and design programs with little sensitivity to local concerns. Too often, we have viewed the poor as "targets for evangelism" or as "beneficiaries" of our programs. That is intolerable. Just as health development workers must establish a new, collaborative relationship with those whom they want to serve in the community, so western missions must establish a new relationship with the indigenous church. Health development is not a commodity to be delivered but a process to be encouraged through relationships of trust.

12. **The Church empowered** - Our task in health development is to help empower the poor and oppressed to address the problems and issues that prevent them from realizing their full potential. Though created in the image of God, that image has been tarnished by the conditions within which many of the world's poor live. With a proper understanding of salvation, a broader definition of health, and new relationships and new skills, the Church can continue to share the love of Christ to the world—and do so more effectively than ever before.

The Journey Continues

The introduction described this book as a journey. The various chapters and case studies have attempted to suggest the lessons that some have learned through their experience in promoting health among the world's poor. These are not the last word on the subject but rather an invitation to dialogue on the nature of health development. You can participate in this process in several ways.

1. **Information** - Gather all the information you can regarding the problems of health — the nature of the problem, causes of illness, strategies for promoting health, etc.

2. **Reflection** - Share your experiences with other practitioners who are wrestling with the same issues. Discover what they have learned and see what might be applicable to your situation.

3. **Decision** - Evaluate what you have learned through your own experience. Consider the ideas that you have gleaned from this book which might be applicable to your situation. Develop a plan through which you can implement these ideas.

4. **Implementation** - Carry out the suggestions and activities that you have outlined in your action plan.

5. **Evaluation** - Assess the results of your action plan. Evaluate what you will then have learned through these activities.

6. **Documentation** - Record what you have learned through your experience. Prepare a case study or article in order to share this with others who could benefit from your experience.

The task of building better models and more effective strategies for health development is an on-going process of reflection and action. We must learn from what we have done and act upon what we have learned. All of us can contribute to this process by working together, coordinating our efforts, sharing information and encouraging each other. Together, we can learn what it means to be the people of God, promoting health and wholeness throughout the world.

MAP International

MAP International is a non-profit global health organization, a leader in promoting total health care for needy people in the developing world. We work through the Church, supporting and encouraging the health workers already in place, serving those who have dedicated their lives to serving the poor.

Since 1954, MAP has provided over $500 million in donated medicines and supplies through 650 mission hospitals and clinics in 80 countries in Africa, Asia and Latin America.

MAP's programs for total health and development include cooperating in experimental community-initiative processes as well as training of health workers and Church leaders through seminars, workshops and on-site consultations in community-building skills, health training, strategy planning and administration.

This monograph is another publication presented by MAP International to the global Christian community to encourage constructive dialog, reflection and action so that, working together, we can have greater effectiveness in proclaiming total health to the world's poor, in Christ's name.

For additional copies of this monograph, a complete publications listing, or more information about MAP International, please contact:

Learning Resource Center
MAP International
P.O. Box 50
Brunswick, GA 31521-0050
U.S.A.
(912) 265-6010